Is COVID-19 a Bioweapon?

A SCIENTIFIC AND FORENSIC INVESTIGATION

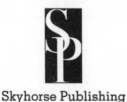

3. A Prion-like Domain at the Receptor Binding Site (RBS).

1. An HIV Pseudovirus glycoprotein 120.

N-Terminal Domain

2. A Proline-Arginine-Arginine-Alanine Insert.

Dr. Richard M. Fleming
PHD, MD, JD

Skyhorse Publishing

Skyhorse Publishing books may be purchased in bulk at special discounts for sales promotion, corporate gifts, fund-raising, or educational purposes. Special editions can also be created to specifications. For details, contact the Special Sales Department, Skyhorse Publishing, 307 West 36th Street, 11th Floor, New York, NY 10018 or info@skyhorsepublishing.com.

Skyhorse® and Skyhorse Publishing® are registered trademarks of Skyhorse Publishing, Inc.®, a Delaware corporation.

Visit our website at www.skyhorsepublishing.com.

10 9 8 7 6 5 4 3

Library of Congress Cataloging-in-Publication Data is available on file.

Print ISBN: 978-1-5107-7019-5
Ebook ISBN: 978-1-5107-7020-1

Printed in the United States of America

Contents

Foreword   iv

Chapter 1. What Is Gain-of-Function Research?   1

Chapter 2. Peter Daszak of EcoHealth, Ralph S. Baric, and
   Shi Zhengli-Li   11

Chapter 3. The Paper Trail of the US Funding for Gain-
   of-Function Research   27

Chapter 4. The SARS-CoV-2 Gain-of-Function Smoking Gun
   Is the Spike Protein   89

Chapter 5. An Intentionally Released Bioweapon   101

The Interview   105

Conclusion: A Gain-of-Function Bioweapon   133

Appendix   137

Endnotes   145

Foreword

By 1999, US federal agencies were funding Gain-of-Function research. In fact, research records reach back decades before that show intentional and knowing efforts to alter viruses. The available published papers strongly suggest that this research is, by its very nature, designed to increase the ability of pathogens to infect and harm people. In 2019, one of those pathogens was intentionally released upon the world in a Wuhan, China wet market. The key to proving and understanding this bioweapon is its spike protein, the very same spike protein being made in millions of people after the COVID-19 vaccines are injected into them. These vaccines are nothing more than the genetic code of this bioweapon. The research publications, patent publications, and grant money trail reveal who is ultimately criminally responsible for the design and development of this weapon, a weapon that violates the Biological Weapons Convention (BWC) treaty, exposing those who have committed crimes against humanity!

For those of you reading this book, a quick search of the internet might lead you to initially think you shouldn't believe what I say. But dig deeper, and you will discover the real truth about my struggles with big pharma, the Food and Drug Administration, and the Department of Health and Human Services. Interestingly, these are the very same organizations who funded the development of this Gain-of-Function bioweapon.

For those of you who have the feeling that something isn't quite right, I encourage you to read what they don't want you to read, and know what they don't want you to know: what they don't want you to know is *the truth*!

* * *

Once you've read and listened to the truth, then you have to make a decision. Do you take the blue pill so you can continue to believe that everything is as it should be? That the courts, attorneys, politicians, scientists, and doctors are all good and just people truly looking out for you? Or do you decide to take the red pill and discover *the truth*? Understand that once you choose the red pill and read this book, there's no going back.

Let me make one final statement before we delve into the facts and evidence showing the Gain-of-Function research and development of this spike protein and bioweapon. I want to make it perfectly clear that by myself this information would not have been possible. The cost of this information is not trivial. Many people have risked their safety and possibly their lives, so that all of us may be the beneficiaries of the extensive research brought forward in this book. They know who they are, and rather than expose them and place them at further risk, I simply want to recognize them here and now. To them, we owe a debt of gratitude that cannot easily be repaid. There are yet others who stood firm against the misinformation being promulgated—against me and against you. These people took on the challenge of helping to bring this information to light, and while I will not expose them for the same reasons, we all owe them a debt of gratitude as well.

> *All truths are easy to understand once they are discovered; the point is to discover them.*
>
> —Galileo Galilei

One Additional Thought

While the information in this book might seem a little overwhelming at first glance, the purpose of this book is not to turn you into an expert on viruses, research, or medicine. The detail has been put here to lay to rest *any* questions about where the virus came from and who was involved in making it. Incontrovertible evidence will be brought forth in this book to uncover those responsible for violating the Biological Weapons Convention treaty, the Nuremberg Code, or the International Covenant on Civil and Political Rights (ICCPR) treaty.

This book is designed to expose once and for all those criminally responsible for the bioweapon known as SARS-CoV-2, the virus that causes COVID-19. This book is designed for you. So when someone questions you or calls you a conspiracy theorist, you can take this book, hand it to him or her, and say, "Here's your proof."

This time there will be no pulling the wool over the jury's eyes . . . This time the world is going to see the real evidence—it will no longer be hidden!!!

CHAPTER 1

What Is Gain-of-Function Research?

Beginning in 2019, most of us became familiar with a new virus. This virus was called SARS-CoV-2 (which can cause the disease called COVID-19). For most people, this virus infected either the lungs or gastrointestinal (GI) track and resolved—or at least we thought so—but as the virus spread around the world a new sense of fear and panic engulfed the world. Amid the chaos, hospital systems became overwhelmed, people began to die from the associated InflammoThrombotic Response (ITR) precipitated by this viral infection, people and societies shut down and broke down, and economies went into a free fall. People surrendered personal freedoms in exchange for perceived security. Families and nations became sharply divided, while governments implemented executive orders replacing elected officials with administratively appointed doctrine equivalent to the Enabling Act[1] of 1933.

My involvement with SARS-CoV-2 began in January 2020. In reality, it began more than a quarter of a century before when I introduced the Inflammation and Heart Disease theory at the sixty-seventh American Heart Association Scientific Sessions in November 1994. This theory was reexplained the following year at a variety of scientific conferences around the world, eventually being published in a cardiology textbook in 1999.[2] Also beginning in 1999, following my discovery of misinformation promulgated by nuclear imaging isotope companies, I began development of the first quantitative method for imaging the body and measuring regional blood flow and metabolism changes. This test not only provided for reductions in the amount of nuclear imaging isotopes given to patients but made it possible to accurately, consistently, and reproducibly measure these differences in the body, allowing for differentiation of changes going on in the body—changes that would become necessary to measure this virus and its response to treatments. By 2017, I had fully developed and patented the Fleming Method for Tissue and Vascular Differentiation and Metabolism (FMTVDM).[3]

During January 2020, I began my work with SARS-CoV-2 by investigating what drugs—based upon published research on other viruses—might have a beneficial treatment effect on this virus, including attacking the ability of the virus to infect cells and reproduce itself, as well as stopping or at least reducing the inflammation and blood clotting (InflammoThrombotic Response) caused by the immune response to the virus in people with comorbidities.[4]

Like others, I soon realized we had entered a new era in human history, when the healthy were being quarantined and tested, medications were being denied to those who were infected or hospitalized, ventilators were being used incorrectly[5] for the level of inflammation present in the lungs, and vaccines were being touted as the only possible solution to the virus.

Like many of you, I began to ask questions, and the answers I found lead to more questions about the ultimate motives of the people involved. For patients becoming infected and those being hospitalized, we had turned the practice of medicine and honest scientific investigation over to the government and those funded by the government, just as the German Medical Association and scientists of the day had turned it over to Adolf Hitler.[6] Germany would later apologize for the action, but it would be too little, too late.[7]

Despite the Nuremberg Code of 1947 and the International Covenant on Civil and Political Rights (ICCPR) treaty being implemented in an effort to prevent such atrocities being committed by people upon people ever again, we find ourselves in the same situation today—unethical experiments[8] conducted by those in power upon those not in power. When the government[9] is involved in experimentation on its citizens, it must use a combination of fear and hope to effectively control the people and manipulate them into submission. What follows is the information about those in power and their experimentation using viruses to infect and harm people using Gain-of-Function.

THE STORY OF GAIN-OF-FUNCTION

As mentioned in the foreword, around 1999, the US Department of Health and Human Services (HHS) began funding research looking at infectious diseases. This research included looking at how such infections might become more infective. One of the original proposed premises behind this type of research, known as Gain-of-Function, was to better understand how something like a coronavirus might mutate over time. If such mutations were to occur, such investigation might allow physicians and scientists an opportunity to stay ahead of such infections. However, what began as observation soon became something altogether different. Instead of asking questions about what might happen naturally, this research become one of intentionally making those changes occur, not in small incremental steps as might occur naturally, but in larger steps that would most likely take centuries to occur—if at all.

In April 2000 while working at the Carolina Vaccine Institute at the University of North Carolina, Ralph S. Baric had already successfully used reverse genetics[10] to generate a chimeric[11] (Gain-of-Function) coronavirus. He not only published[12] this research funded by the NIH (grant numbers AI23946, GM63228, and AI26603) but also received a patent[13] for it in 2003:

> This approach facilitates the reconstruction of genomes and chromosomes in Vitro for reintroduction into a living host, and allows the Selected mutagenesis and genetic manipulation of Sequences in Vitro prior to reassembly into a full length genome molecule for reintroduction into the same or different host. (United States Patent No. US006593111B2)

In 2002 following the SARS-CoV-1 outbreak in China, Dr. Shi Zhengli, a.k.a. Shi Zhengli-Li, and colleagues at the Wuhan Institute of Virology (WIV) began investigating how SARS-CoV-1 was transmitted.[14] In particular, Zhengli was interested in how SARS-CoV-1 could be transmitted from person to person. To do this, she developed chimeric (Gain-of-Function) coronaviruses using human immunodeficiency virus-based pseudovirus[15] systems with the cell lines of people, civet cats, and horseshoe bats.

In March 2004, HHS announced that it was going to create the National Science Advisory Board for Biosecurity (NSABB) to be managed by the National Institutes of Health (NIH). A press release[16] issued by then Secretary of HHS Thompson states the following:

> Our nation has been a world leader in life sciences research because of our emphasis on the importance of the free flow of scientific inquiry. **Yet, sadly,**

the very same tools developed to better the health and condition of humankind can also be used for its destruction. [Emphasis added.]

In 2005, Baric published a paper—omitting unpublished research (p. 21 in Baric's paper)—declaring he could alter the genome of coronaviruses, noting the "alteration of any part of the coronavirus genome."[17]

In 2006, using chimeric (Gain-of-Function) research, Chinese scientists reported their ability to combine parts of four different viruses into a single viral genome.[18] This report raises a few serious questions in my mind.

First, why were these researchers combining parts of four dangerous viruses—specifically, hepatitis C virus (HCV), human immunodeficiency virus -1 (HIV-1), SARS-CoV-1 (identified as SARS-CoV-1 and not SARS-CoV), and SARS-CoV-2?

Second, if as we've been told, SARS-CoV-2 didn't appear until 2019 and there were no identified naturally occurring SARS-CoV-2 reported between this 2006 publication and 2019, then doesn't this at least in part suggest that SARS-CoV-2 is not naturally occurring but man-made?

Third, if the answer to question number two is that the virus is man-made, going as far back as 2006, then doesn't this add credence to those who have cautioned that SARS-CoV-1 was a bioweapon and SARS-CoV-2 is an upgraded version of that bioweapon?

Finally, looking at the much-talked-about number of cycles used for polymerase chain reaction (PCR) verification of the presence of these viruses, and taking into consideration what Kary Mullis recommended for cutoffs for PCR cycles when he submitted and received his patent for PCR (see chapter 2), why were the cycles used for detection of SARS-CoV-2 set so high by the FDA?[19]

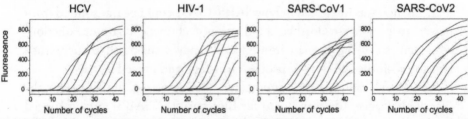

Fig. 1. Calibration of the real-time RT-PCR assay for HCV, HIV-1, SARS-CoV1, and SARS-CoV2.

We diluted purified and calibrated armored RNA with pooled normal human plasma supplemented with 1 g/L sodium azide and prepared 200-μL aliquots by 10-fold serial dilution to obtain samples containing 10^{10} to 10^1 copies. From these materials, we isolated template RNA ranging from 10^{10} to 10^1 copies (from *left* to *right*) for RT-PCR assays. Water was used as a negative control. All RNA templates were assayed in a single run using a diagnostic reagent set (Intec) for each individual virus. Real-time RT-PCR was conducted on an iCycler iQ thermal cycler (Bio-Rad).

By 2007, the US government must have had sufficient questions about the potential for a pandemic—sufficient at least for the government to fund research to address their questions. In that year, research funded by a National Science Foundation (NSF) award IIS-0513650 and the European Commission (contract 001907) was published, addressing the critical need to shut down international travel for containment purposes should an emerging disease raise concerns about global spread—that is, a pandemic.[20]

The questions are, why wasn't this Dr. Anthony S. Fauci's recommendation to President Trump when pandemic concerns were first raised, and why did it fall to a politician to make the right decision when there was published scientific research paid for by the US government to answer the question about shutting down international travel?

Concerns from the scientific community about Gain-of-Function research began to be front-page news around 2011 when Gain-of-Function H5N1 lethal Asian Influenza Virus (a.k.a. bird flu) was released from labs in the Netherlands and the University of Wisconsin.[21] The National Institute of Allergy and Infectious Diseases (NIAID) supported the H5N1 influenza transmissible studies conducted by Dr. Yoshihiro Kawaoka at the University of Wisconsin and Dr. Ron Fouchier at Erasmus Medical Center in the Netherlands.

The Centers for Disease Control and Prevention (CDC) has admitted[22] that the CDC also has been involved in Gain-of-Function research with the "highly pathogenic avian influenza A (H5N1) virus."[23] This H5N1 research included reverse genetics and the Laboratory of Infectious Diseases, NIAID.[24] Genetic reassortment used in this research is the mixing of genetic material of a species into new combinations.

On April 26, 2012, Dr. Fauci testified before the Committee on Homeland Security and Governmental Affairs of the United States Senate on "Dual Use Research of Concern: Balancing Benefits and Risks" as the director for the NIAID, National Institutes of Health, US Department of Health and Human Services. He was called to address the concerns regarding the NIAID-supported H5N1 influenza transmissible studies conducted by Dr. Yoshihiro Kawaoka[25] at the University of Wisconsin and Dr. Ron Fouchier at Erasmus Medical Center in the Netherlands and the lethal threat posed by this Gain-of-Function research.

Dr. Fauci established early in his presentation that NIAID was involved in such Dual Use Research of Drs. Kawaoka and Fouchier, stating the H5N1 influenza transmissibility studies were "NIAID-supported." Dual

Use Research is the term used when it is understood that such research might be intended for benefit but might also be easily misapplied to do harm.

Regarding such research, there are very specific questions[26] researchers were asked, including the following:

Can the research be reasonably anticipated to produce one or more of the seven experimental effects/categories listed below?

1. Will an intermediate or final product of your research make a vaccine less effective or ineffective? Yes/No
2. Will the final or intermediate product of your research confer resistance to antibiotics or antivirals in ways that are inherently different than those published previously? Yes/No
3. Will your work enhance the virulence of a pathogen or render a nonpathogen virulent? Yes/No
4. Will the results of your work increase the transmissibility of any pathogen? Yes/No
5. Will your research result in alteration of the host range of a pathogen? Yes/No
6. Will your research result in a product or intermediate that that may prevent or interfere with diagnosis of infection or disease? Yes/No
7. Does your research enable "weaponization" of an agent or toxin? Yes/No
8. Even though your research did not involve any of the aforementioned seven criteria, and recognizing that your work product or results of your research could conceivably be misused, is there the potential for your results/product to be readily utilized to cause public harm? Yes/No
   • If the answer is no, no further action is required, but the PI [principle investigator] should conduct an ongoing assessment to be sure this continues to be the case and must file an annual report of that assessment.
   • If one or more of the seven experimental effects/ categories listed above can potentially occur, the Institutional Biosafety Committee (IBC) working with the PI assesses if the criteria defining DURC (Dual Use Research of Concern) would potentially be met. Again if the answer is no, no further action is required, but

the PI should conduct an ongoing assessment to be sure this continues to be the case and must file an annual report of that assessment.

- If the criteria defining DURC would potentially be met, the IBC working with the PI must develop and implement a risk management plan based on the risk assessment. The conduct and/or communication of the research findings must adhere to the risk management plan with ongoing oversight by the IBC with respect to DURC and in consultation with the Intramural Research's Dual Use Committee as appropriate.

Given the specificity of these questions and the admission by Dr. Fauci acknowledging such NIAID funding—along with other federal agencies—for such Gain-of-Function research, it is hard to understand how such Dual Use Gain-of-Function research could repeatedly receive funding.

Since the development of a Gain-of-Function bioweapon is a direct violation of the Biological Weapons Convention (BWC) treaty, it is easy to understand why Senator Dr. Rand Paul and Senator John Kennedy have been so interested in questioning Dr. Fauci about the Gain-of-Function research money he has been responsible for providing to Peter Daszak. Should it be determined that a criminal investigation is required and a special prosecutor be needed, Professor David A. Clements of the University of New Mexico School of Law has offered to fill that role.

The result of this 2012 investigation into Gain-of-Function research resulted in a voluntary moratorium that lasted almost one year and ended in January 2013.[27]

In 2014, Baric and Chinese researchers published a paper demonstrating differences between spike proteins that can infect bats and those capable of infecting people.[28] This research was funded by NIH grants RO1AI089728 and R21AI109094.

In October 2014, only a year after lifting the voluntary moratorium, the Obama Administration placed a ban on Gain-of-Function research[29] after it was discovered that the CDC had accidentally exposed workers to Anthrax and unwittingly shipped out samples of influenza virus contaminated with the deadly H5N1 virus. Meanwhile, the NIH found vials of smallpox in a storeroom: that for fifty years had been unaccounted for.

Finally, in 2015, Zhengli and Baric both announced they had "reengineered" (i.e., Gain-of-Function) the spike protein of coronaviruses so they could infect human cells:

> **reengineered** HKU4 spike, aiming to build its capacity to mediate viral entry into human cells. To this end, we **introduced two single mutations.** . . . Mutations in these motifs in coronavirus spikes have **demonstrated dramatic effects on viral entry into human cells**. [Emphasis added.][30]

This research was paid for by NIH grants RO1AI089728 and RO1AI110700. Following the publication, Shi Zhengli-Li and Ralph S. Baric announced to the world, as reported by scientific journalist Matt Ridley, that they were capable of making more virulent, pathogenic viruses.[31]

Recommendations for the oversight of Gain-of-Function research were made on April 7, 2016, and approved on March 15, 2016, by the National Science Advisory Board for Biosecurity (NSABB). Included in that report on the list of ex officio members is Dr. Anthony S. Fauci (on page 102).[32] Also noted in that report was Speaker/Commenter Ralph Baric, PhD (on page 68).

The Gain-of-Function ban was lifted in December 2017.[33]

By 2019, the November 14, 2018, research presentation made by Zhengli at the Shanghai Jiao Tong University, entitled "Studies on Bat Coronavirus and Its Cross-Specific Infection," was deleted from the university website.

During the summer of 2019, the Wuhan Institute of Virology genetic databank records, including its viral genomes and research, were wiped—months before the recognition of the emergence of SARS-CoV-2. On December 31, 2019, the Wuhan Municipal Health Commission report briefing on what would later be identified as SARS-CoV-2 was also deleted.[34]

Final Thoughts on Gain-of-Function

Research scientists are a particular type of people; I know because I am one. We are driven by an insatiable desire to learn, understand, or find answers to questions we have. Sometimes those questions appear to be of no interest to others, but over the course of time, all knowledge adds together. This addition of knowledge can either be used for good purposes or for not-so-good purposes. Gain-of-Function research is one such area of research where the outcomes can be used for good or evil, depending upon the motives of those involved.

While most people believe that SARS-CoV-2 first appeared in 2019, evidence shows the virus responsible for the InflammoThrombotic disease known as COVID-19 was being manipulated two provinces from Wuhan in 2006, and the work continued forward.[35] Those initial genetic sequences are shown in the appendix. But as you are about to see, the research into Gain-of-Function of this and other biological agents is occurring not merely in China but also around the world—including, I would argue, unfortunately, in the United States of America—and it is being funded by our federal agencies from taxpayer dollars.

As President Eisenhower said in his farewell address (see chapter 3), we need look no further than our own backyard.

CHAPTER 2

Peter Daszak of EcoHealth, Ralph S. Baric, and Shi Zhengli-Li

When research scientists receive grants—particularly from the federal government—they are expected to demonstrate that the money has been used for the purposes for which it was intended. As a result, scientists and physicians are expected to publish the results of that research. These publications leave an indelible mark on history.

Research careers are built upon proving that the work a scientist has completed has advanced the quest for knowledge, and scientists share that information with colleagues—all to advance the sciences.

The founding fathers recognized the importance of such work and granted a US constitutional right to individuals who advance science sufficiently as to produce a new invention deemed useful to humanity. The power to grant patents to inventors falls under the legislative branch of the federal government, also known as Congress. These patents therefore provide an indelible record of what has transpired and by whom.

For these reasons, we will now look at just some of the publication and patent record evidence that SARS-CoV-2, in addition to other viruses, is the result of Gain-of-Function research, with a record in published research, patents, and, as we will see in this and the next chapter, funding.

To promote the Progress of Science and useful Arts, by securing for limited Times to Authors and Inventors the exclusive Right to their respective Writings and Discoveries

—US Constitution, Article I, Section 8, § 8.

1974: The First Known Manmade Altered Virus

To the best of my knowledge, the first[1] reported genetically altered (Gain-of-Function) virus was the Qß phage in 1974.[2] This Gain-of-Function research—like many of the projects that followed these investigators—was paid for by Federal NIH Research Project (ROI) grants.

1985: Baric's Early Work with Recombination of Coronaviruses

To the best of my knowledge, Ralph Baric began working with coronaviruses found in mice back in the mid-1980s. In 1985, while at the University of California, Los Angeles (UCLA), he and colleagues at the University of Texas Health Science Center at Houston (UTHSCH) conducted research on recombinant viruses, including coronaviruses.[3] This research was paid for by a variety of grants, including the National Science Foundation (PCM-4507) and US Public Health research grant (AI 19244). US Public Health is a division of the US Department of Health and Human Services (HHS).

1987: Patent granted to Dr. Kary B. Mullis for Polymerase Chain Reaction (PCR)

Patent number 4,683,195 was granted to Mullis and others for "a process for detecting the presence or absence of at least one specific nucleic acid sequence in a sample containing a nucleic acid or mixture of nucleic acids."

A clear review of this patent shows that Mullis did not exceed fifteen to twenty cycles[4] of PCR for the identification of genetic material.

	Number of Double Strands After 0 to n Cycles		
Cycle Number	Template	Long Products	Specific Sequence [S]
1	1	1	0
2	1	2	1
3	1	3	4
5	1	5	26
10	1	10	1013
15	1	15	32,752
20	1	20	1,048,555
n	1	n	$(2^n - n - 1)$

1994: Fleming Introduces the Inflammation and Heart Disease Theory

In 1994 at the American Heart Association meetings, I first presented my Theory on Inflammation and Heart Disease. I would repeat my presentation in 1995, and, by 1999, my theory would become part of a cardiology textbook.[5] The schematic of this theory is shown in the appendix. The theory, which explains the inflammation and thrombotic chronic diseases,[6] would later go on to be discussed on *20/20*[7] and other programs. I published the role of many factors—including bacteria and viruses—involved in producing both inflammation and blood clotting, a process I have since referred to as InflammoThrombotic Response (ITR). It is this ITR that is responsible for COVID-19 and the deaths resulting from individuals not treated for the ITR.[8]

2000: Making DNA from RNA—Reverse Transcription: Lessons Learned from HIV

In early 2000, we know that researchers in Spain, whose work was communicated by Paul Ahlquist from the University of Wisconsin, showed how combining complementary DNA (cDNA) with nuclear expression of RNA allowed the researchers to develop a synthetic virus.[9] Complementary DNA is a single-stranded DNA molecule that is chemically made from single-stranded RNA. To do this requires an enzyme called *reverse transcriptase* (RT). RT makes it possible for the cDNA to be made from the RNA. During the engineering of this infectious cDNA virus, the spike protein of the virus was replaced with the spike protein genes from another virus. The result was a chimeric (Gain-of-Function) virus that infected the gastrointestinal system of pigs. The researchers concluded this could now be used for dogs, cats, and people:

> This cDNA may also be the basis for a tissue-specific expression system that may be used in four species—human, porcine, canine, and feline—by replacing the S gene included in the cDNA with that of the coronavirus infecting the target species. It is anticipated that by this procedure either fully infectious viruses or at least partially competent isolates able to express foreign genes will be generated, both being of practical interest.[10]

2000: Making an Infective Transmissible Virus

Following funding from NIH (Grant AI 239476), Baric and others "enhanced" a transmissible gastroenteritis virus (TGEV):

> The availability of TGEV infectious constructs will obviously benefit studies of all aspects of TGEV biology and pathogenesis, including analysis of the coronavirus replicase and the somewhat controversial transcription processes which govern expression of the subgenome-length mRNAs (17, 40, 42, 43).[11]

The infection produced by the synthetically (human) made cDNA was indistinguishable from the infectious wild-type virus, as noted by Baric:

> These data indicate that viruses derived from the infectious cDNA construct had phenotypes **indistinguishable** from those of wild-type TGEV in swine cells. [Emphasis added.][12]

From this research it is clear that Baric and others foresaw the potential to further manipulate/engineer DNA:

> Our approach, however, may provide a means to address the function of large blocks of DNA, like pathogenesis islands, or to directly engineer chromosomes that contain large gene cassettes of interest (12).

2001: Others Demonstrate the Ability to Generate Coronaviruses Using Recombinant (Genetic) Engineering

In 2001, a group of German researchers showed that they too could produce an infectious coronavirus using a vaccinia virus.[13] (*Vaccina* is a linear double-stranded DNA virus. It is the source of the modern smallpox vaccine.) These researchers not only showed that they could produce an infectious coronavirus but also that they could recover it in MRC-5 cells (a type of cells that allow researchers recovery).[14]

To make a recombinant organism, the gene of interest must first be isolated and removed using restriction enzymes.[15] These enzymes work like "molecular scissors" to cut the DNA on both sides of the gene of interest. The DNA fragment is then ligated (joined) into the DNA of a vector.

The researchers noted the benefit of this reverse-genetics approach:

> Classical approach can now be complemented by a **reverse-genetic** approach. Moreover, the system we describe also facilitates, in principle, the analysis of

coronavirus replication, independent of the virus life-cycle and **without the requirement for receptor mediated infection**. Thus, it can be put to great advantage in the analysis of the virus-host cell interaction in the context of virus replication, transcription, assembly and release.

Secondly, the system we describe will complement existing methods of producing recombinant coronaviruses (Masters, 1999; Almazán et al., 2000; Yount et al., 2000) and significantly advance the **analysis of coronavirus pathogenesis**. With the systems now available, **it should be possible to generate rapidly a large collection of genetically modified coronaviruses**; for example, intra- and interspecific **chimeric viruses**, viruses with **gene inactivations or deletions** and viruses with **attenuating modifications or supplementary functions**. The phenotypes associated with these modifications, at least those that are not lethal, can then be tested in animal models of infection. In particular, this should provide **important insights** into the relationship between **coronavirus infection** and **the immune response**.

Finally, the results we present should also encourage the development of coronavirus vectors for the expression of heterologous proteins. **In the long term, we believe that the expression of multiple subgenomic mRNAs in coronavirus infected cells could form the basis of a vector system that allows the expression of multiple transcriptional units, each encoding a heterologous protein. These features and the autonomy of coronavirus RNA replication could then be exploited in the development of a new class of RNA vaccine vectors.** (Bredenbeek & Rice, 1992; Mandl et al., 1998)[16] [Emphasis added.]

As you read through the previous paragraphs, I would recommend you pay particular attention to the words I have emphasized. They provide an interesting insight to what we have seen since 2019.

2001: Baric and Colleagues Apply for a Patent to Manipulate Genes

By May 2001, Baric and Yount filed a patent designed to allow them to control and profit from genetic manipulation of plants, animals, bacteria, and viruses—including coronaviruses. The patent was granted on July 15, 2003. This patent included research supported by US taxpayer funding.[17]

US006593111B2

(12) **United States Patent**
     Baric et al.

(10) **Patent No.:**   **US 6,593,111 B2**
(45) **Date of Patent:**   **Jul. 15, 2003**

(54) **DIRECTIONAL ASSEMBLY OF LARGE VIRAL GENOMES AND CHROMOSOMES**

(75) Inventors: **Ralph S. Baric**, Haw River, NC (US); **Boyd Yount**, Hillsborough, NC (US)

(73) Assignee: **University of North Carolina at Chapel Hill**, Chapel Hill, NC (US)

(*) Notice: Subject to any disclaimer, the term of this patent is extended or adjusted under 35 U.S.C. 154(b) by 0 days.

(21) Appl. No.: **09/862,847**

(22) Filed: **May 21, 2001**

(65)   **Prior Publication Data**

US 2002/0177230 A1 Nov. 28, 2002

Related U.S. Application Data

(60) Provisional application No. 60/206,537, filed on May 21, 2000, and provisional application No. 60/285,320, filed on Apr. 20, 2001.

(51) Int. Cl.[7] **C12P 21/06**; C12N 7/00
(52) U.S. Cl. **435/69.1**; 435/235.1; 536/23.72
(58) Field of Search 435/69.1, 235.1; 536/23.72

(56)   **References Cited**

U.S. PATENT DOCUMENTS

5,202,430 A   4/1993   Brian et al. 536/23.72
5,916,570 A   6/1999   Kapil 424/222.1

Lai, Michael M.C. "The making of infectious viral RNA: No size limit in sight," *PNAS*. vol. 97, No. 10, May 9, 2000, pp. 5025–5027.

Almazan et al., "Engineering the largest RNA virus genome as an infectious bacterial artificial chromosome," *Proceedings of the National Academy of Sciences of USA* 97: 5516–5521 (2000).

Thiel et al., "Infectious RNA transcribed in vitro from a cDNA copy of the human coronavirus genome cloned in vaccinia virus," 82: 1273–1281 (2001).

Yount et al., "Strategy for systematic assembly of large RNA and DNa enomes: Transmissible gastroenteritis virus model," 74: 10600–10611 (2000).

International Search Report of PCT/US01/16564 dated Dec. 7, 2002.

Primary Examiner—Hankyel T. Park
(74) *Attorney, Agent, or Firm*—Myers Bigel Sibley & Sajovec, P.A.

(57)   **ABSTRACT**

Full-length, functionally intact genomes or chromosomes are directionally assembled with partial cDNA or DNA subclones of a genome. This approach facilitates the reconstruction of genomes and chromosomes in vitro for reintroduction into a living host, and allows the selected mutagenesis and genetic manipulation of sequences in vitro prior to reassembly into a full length genome molecule for reintroduction into the same or different host. This approach also provides an alternative to recombination-mediated techniques to manipulate the genomes of higher plants and animals as well as bacteria and viruses.

2003: Making a Coronavirus

In 2003, Baric and others published research[18] funded by NIH grants AI23946, GM63228, and AI26603, showing they could "rescue" SARS-CoV Urbani viruses by using reverse genetics.[19] By taking segments of cDNA and overlapping them, they could fully clone SARS viruses. These clones were then shown to be able to infect VeroE6 cells.[20]

When the N (the nucleocapsid) transcripts were included, greater infection occurred. When cells were not infected by this coronavirus (control cells)—no antibody staining to the virus is seen.

This same research showed that cysteine proteinase inhibitors could prevent cells from being infected. It also indicated that researchers could manipulate the genes of the virus, according to the researchers:

> The current data indicate that the cysteine proteinase inhibitor E64-d may inhibit SARS virus replication at any time during infection. . . . The availability of a full-length cDNA of the SARS genome should allow for genetic manipulation of the replicase gene providing new insights into the role of specific proteolytic cleavages and replicase proteins during viral replication.[21]

The first part of this conclusion to their research clearly demonstrated an interest in further genetic manipulation of the virus. The later part is critical to understanding the ability to treat SARS-CoV-2. The targeting of this transmembrane protease serine 2 by clindamycin is one of the reasons why I chose to include this in the treatment of patients infected with SARS-CoV-2, and those experiencing the InflammoThrombotic Response (ITR) known as COVID-19.[22]

Not only does the nucleocapsid (N) structural protein of SARS viruses appear to play a significant role in increasing infectivity, but also, for SARS-CoV-2, it has been shown to insert (reverse transcribe) its genetic sequence into the human DNA—once again funded by NIH grants (1U19AI131135-01, 5R01MH104610-21). This reverse transcription (RT) has since been shown to occur in all but three of the twenty-three pairs of human chromosomes.[23]

2006: Chimeric (Gain-of-Function) cDNA made from HCV, HIV-1, SARS-CoV-1, and SARS-CoV-2

In 2006, Chinese researchers spliced four target cDNA segments together to form a single 1,200-nucleotide-long RNA sequence.[24] This chimeric (Gain-of-Function) sequence included combining hepatitis C virus (HCV), human immunodeficiency virus – 1 (HIV-1), SARS-CoV-1, and SARS-CoV-2. This genetic sequence is shown in the appendix. This research was funded by the Fujian[25] government (Grant number 2003Y004).

2007: SARS-CoV (SARS-CoV-1) Genome[26] Patent Assigned to US Department of Health & Human Services

In May 2007, a patent was granted for isolation of human SARS-CoV-1.[27] The assignee—the party that would profit financially from the patent—was the US Department of Health and Human Services (HHS). This isolation not only genetically identified the virus but also established the polymerase chain reaction (PCR) test to find SARS-CoV-1. In April 2020, the FDA issued an umbrella Emergency Use Authorization (EUA) for PCR testing of SARS-CoV-2.[28]

2007: Research Shows Insertions Placed in Spike Proteins Makes It Possible for SARS-CoV to Infect Human Cells

Research published by Dr. Zhengli and researchers at the Australian Animal Health Laboratory looked at SARS-like coronaviruses (SL-CoVs) found in horseshoe bats and SARS-associated coronavirus (SARS-CoV).[29] While they found a significant amount of similar genetic material, they also discovered that SL-CoVs could *not* bind to human ACE2 receptors. Zhengli and the other scientists discovered that the SL-CoV spike protein was unable to use ACE2 receptors to infect human cells. However, if they inserted amino acids not naturally found in these viruses, at the N-terminal domain through Gain-of-Function (chimeric) manipulation, they discovered they could produce viruses able to infect human cells.

2010: Shi Zhengli-Li Conducts Chimeric Experiments Showing SARS-CoV Spike Protein Unable to Bind to ACE2 Human Cell Receptors

In 2010, Shi Zhengli conducted chimeric research on SARS-CoV-1 (then called SARS-CoV), including combining HIV-pseudovirus to look at the binding capacity of this virus with human ACE2 receptors.[30] Their work specifically included altering (through mutagenesis) the spike proteins to determine how to increase the spike protein binding to the ACE2 receptor.

The research showed no proline-arginine-arginine-alanine (PRRA)[31] insert critical to the binding of the SARS-CoV-2 to ACE2 receptors on human cells. As noted in this published research (jointly done by Dr. Zhengli at the Wuhan Institute of Virology, researchers in Australia, and the University of Minnesota Medical School), not only is the spike protein from horseshoe bats unable to bind to ACE2 receptors, but also these differences along with differences in civets[32] highlight a critical missing piece to the zoonotic theory of the original of SARS-CoV-2:

> However, although the genetically related SARS-like coronavirus (SL-CoV) has been identified in horseshoe bats of the genus Rhinolophus [5, 8, 12, 18], **its spike protein was not able to use the human ACE2 (hACE2) protein as a receptor**. Close examination of the crystal structure of human SARS-CoV RBD complexed with hACE2 suggests that truncations in the receptor-binding motif (RBM) region of SL-CoV spike protein abolish its hACE2-binding ability [7, 10], and hence the SL-CoV found recently in horseshoe bats is unlikely to be the direct ancestor of human SARS-CoV.

Also, it has been shown that **the human SARS-CoV spike protein and its closely related civet SARS-CoV spike protein were not able to use a horseshoe bat** (R. pearsoni) ACE2 as a receptor [13], **highlighting a critical missing link in the bat-to-civet/human transmission** chain of SARSCoV. [Emphasis added.]

2013: SARS-CoV Associated with Lethal Blood Clotting in the Lungs

Baric and people working with him discovered in 2013 that SARS-CoV—in research funded by NIAID, NIH, the National Center for Advancing Translational Sciences (NIH/NCATS), and HHS (grants HHSN272200800060C; 5UL1RR024140)—had four critical genes that were expressed following SARS-CoV infections:

The results of these studies demonstrate that a fine balance exists between host coagulation and fibrinolysin pathways regulating pathological disease outcomes, including diffuse alveolar damage and acute lung injury, following infection with highly pathogenic respiratory viruses, such as SARS-CoV.[33]

They went on to show that this was critical to infection and lung damage:

The urokinase pathway had a significant effect on both lung pathology and overall SARS-CoV pathogenesis.

As the lung tissue slides from the research showed, the larger the viral load (greater infection), the greater the damage to the lungs with fibrin (blood clotting).[34]

2014: Baric Applies for an International Patent to Alter the Spike Protein of Coronaviruses

In March 2014, Professor Baric applied for an international patent for the Methods and Compositions for Chimeric (Gain-of-Function) Coronavirus Spike Proteins. As noted in the next figure, this invention (patent) was made with the support of NIH Grant U54AI057157, which further demonstrated that the US federal government was funding Gain-of-Function research of the coronavirus spike protein.

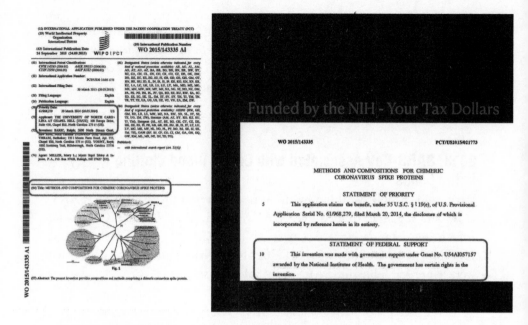

August 2014: Baric Uncovers TMPRSS2[35] Link to Infectivity of MERS

In August 2014, while investigating Middle East Respiratory Syndrome coronavirus (MERS-CoV or MERS), Baric and other researchers from Shanghai University and the University of Minnesota compared MERS with two closely related coronaviruses known as HKU4 and HKU5. Despite some similarities, Baric and others showed that the spike proteins of HKU4 and HKU5[36] do not attach to and infect human cells. However, MERS spike protein specifically attaches to a cellular receptor found in humans known as dipeptidyl peptidase 4 (DPP4).[37]

DPP4 is also known as adenosine deaminase complexing protein 2 or cluster of differentiation 26 (CD26). Stimulating DPP4 results in an immune response and the release of inflammatory cytokines.[38] Like the ACE2 receptor gene, DPP4 is also found on the X-chromosome, further explaining some of the differences between men and women in SARS-CoV-2 infections.[39]

The failure of MERS to bind to ACE2 receptors was confirmed by Chinese researchers in 2020.[40] That leads us to information provided by Dr. Li Meng Yan, namely that SARS-CoV-1[41] was a genetically modified (Gain-of-Function) virus that was also a bioweapon developed by the Chinese Communist Party (CCP), with SARS-CoV-2 being the upgraded version of this bioweapon.[42]

2015: Baric and Zhengli-Li Combine the Backbone of One Virus and the Spike Protein of Another

In June of 2015, both Shi Zhengli-Li and Ralph S. Baric—who had received funding from Peter Daszak of EcoHealth Alliance, along with NIH funding (reviewed and approved)—announced they had used reverse genetics[43] to generate a chimeric (formed from parts of various animals) virus:

> Using the SARS-CoV reverse genetics system, we generated and characterized a chimeric virus expressing the spike of bat coronavirus SHC014 in a mouse-adapted SARS-CoV backbone.[44]

And according to Baric:

> This virus is highly pathogenic, and treatments developed against the original SARS virus in 2002 and the ZMapp drugs used to fight Ebola fail to neutralize and control this particular virus.[45]

While the original publication acknowledged funding for this research from NIH, NIAID[46] and the National Natural Science Foundation of China, and researchers from the Wuhan Institute of Virology, the University of North Carolina, and the University of Texas Medical Branch, the original publication by Baric and others failed to disclose the funding they received from Peter Daszak's EcoHealth Alliance, the United States Agency for International Development (USAID), and the US Central Intelligence Agency (CIA). On November 20, 2015, this omission was corrected and *Nature Medicine* posted a corrigendum[47] (correction with additional information) showing that the funding for this research came from USAID and the CIA:

> In the version of this article initially published online, the authors omitted to acknowledge a funding source, USAID-EPT-PREDICT funding from EcoHealth Alliance, to Z.-L.S. The error has been corrected for the print, PDF and HTML versions of this article.[48]

The supplementary[49] material to this research published by Zhengli-Li and Baric shows that the spike protein of the SHC014-CoV (SL-COV)[50] virus that infects horseshoe bats **was combined with** the backbone of SARS-CoV mouse adapted (MA15) backbone. In addition to combining the spike protein from one virus with the backbone of another virus, Baric and Zhengli-Li inserted (changed) four nucleotides in Open Reading Frame 1a (ORD1a) and Open Reading Frame 1b (ORF1b) of the viral genome.

These nucleotide changes are shown in the following figure.[51] These insertions change the replication proteins required to make this chimeric (Gain-of-Function) virus. A fifth nucleotide change is found at position 26428 in the Envelope Protein,[52] a change found to be important for the SARS-CoV-2 virus to cross the blood-brain barrier, after which the virus can infect and damage the brain.

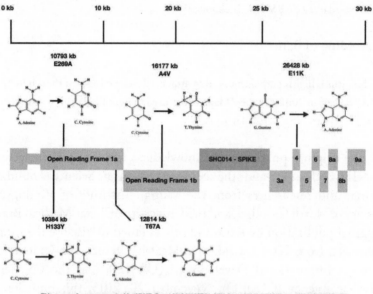

This research was supported by NIAID Grant U19AI109761, NIH Grant U19AI107810, and USAID-PREDICT funding from EcoHealth Alliance to Ralph S. Baric, Ralph S. Baric, and Shi Zhengli-Li respectively.

The research—as noted in the next figure—was funded by the NIAID, NIH, USAID, and EcoHealth Alliance. It specifically states that this Gain-of-Function (GOF) research was reviewed and approved by the NIH and shows funding for both Baric (R.S.B.) and Zhengli-Li Shi (Z.-L.S.).

ACKNOWLEDGMENTS

Research in this manuscript was supported by grants from the National Institute of Allergy & Infectious Disease and the National Institute of Aging of the US National Institutes of Health (NIH) under awards U19AI109761 (R.S.B.), U19AI107810 (R.S.B.), AI085524 (W.A.M.), F32AI102561 (V.D.M.) and K99AG049092 (V.D.M.), and by the National Natural Science Foundation of China awards 81290341 (Z.-L.S.) and 31470260 (X.-Y.G.), and by USAID-EPT-PREDICT funding from EcoHealth Alliance (Z.-L.S.). Human airway epithelial cultures were supported by the National Institute of Diabetes and Digestive and Kidney Disease of the NIH under award NIH DK065988 (S.H.R.). We also thank M.T. Ferris (Dept. of Genetics, University of North Carolina) for the reviewing of statistical approaches and C.T. Tseng (Dept. of Microbiology and Immunology, University of Texas Medical Branch) for providing Calu-3 cells. Experiments with the full-length and chimeric SHC014 recombinant viruses were initiated and performed before the GOF research funding pause and have since been reviewed and approved for continued study by the NIH. The content is solely the responsibility of the authors and does not necessarily represent the official views of the NIH.

AUTHOR CONTRIBUTIONS

V.D.M. designed, coordinated and performed experiments, completed analysis and wrote the manuscript. B.L.Y. designed the infectious clone and recovered chimeric viruses; S.A. completed neutralization assays; L.E.G. helped perform mouse experiments; T.S. and J.A.P. completed mouse experiments and plaque assays; X.-Y.G. performed pseudotyping experiments; K.D. generated structural figures and predictions; E.F.D. generated phylogenetic analysis; R.L.G. completed RNA analysis; S.H.R. provided primary HAE cultures; A.L. and W.A.M. provided critical monoclonal antibody reagents; and Z.-L.S. provided SHC014 spike sequences and plasmids. R.S.B. designed experiments and wrote manuscript.

COMPETING FINANCIAL INTERESTS

In the abstract of this published research, Zhengli-Li and Baric specifically state they have produced a Gain-of-Function (chimeric) virus:

> Using the SARS-CoV reverse genetics system, we generated and characterized a chimeric virus expressing the spike of bat coronavirus SHC014 in a mouse-adapted SARS-CoV backbone.[53]

Zhengli and Baric then go on to state:

> Additionally, in vivo experiments demonstrate replication of the chimeric virus in mouse lung with notable pathogenesis. Evaluation of available SARS-based immune-therapeutic and prophylactic modalities revealed poor efficacy; both monoclonal antibody and vaccine approaches failed to neutralize and protect from infection with CoVs using the novel spike protein. On the

basis of these findings, we synthetically re-derived an infectious full-length SHC014 recombinant virus and demonstrate robust viral replication both in vitro and in vivo.

In the end, the authors (Baric and Zhengli-Li) concluded they had built a more pathogenic virus:

> Thus, relative to the Urbani spike–MA15 CoV, SHC014-MA15 shows a gain in pathogenesis (Fig. 1). **On the basis of these findings, scientific review panels may deem similar studies building chimeric viruses based on circulating strains too risky to pursue, as increased pathogenicity in mammalian models cannot be excluded.** Coupled with restrictions on mouse-adapted strains and the development of monoclonal antibodies using escape mutants, research into CoV emergence and therapeutic efficacy may be severely limited moving forward. Together, these data and restrictions represent a crossroads of GOF research concerns; the potential to prepare for and mitigate future outbreaks must be weighed **against the risk of creating more dangerous pathogens.**[54] [Emphasis added.]

Their chimeric (Gain-of-Function) virus was able "to replicate in human airway cultures, cause pathogenesis . . . and escape current therapeutics." In the end, the researchers appeared to be more concerned about what limitations this might pose on future research they wanted to do than the potential harm they might do to mankind.

Many people over the years have decided they knew what was best for humanity. Bill Gates has commented on more than one occasion that the use of clustered regularly interspaced short palindromic repeats (CRISPR) technology would make it possible to "eliminate undesirable genes" and "potentially swap in preferable alternatives"[55]—a concept held by others in history, including Dr. Joseph Mengele:

> Like all doctors in 1930s Germany, Mengele came under Hitler's concept of German medicine that departed from the traditional caregiving role, Marwell explains. The physician's first responsibility was to the nation, not individual patients. As part of the Führer's weltanschauung, doctors were "biological soldiers," committed to ensuring Germany's glorious destiny by "cleansing" the population of "inferior" genetic material.[56]

This perspective seems to permeate today's society.

September 2015: Zhengli and Baric Reengineer (Gain-of-Function) the HKU4 Spike Protein of MERS to Increase Infectivity in Humans

While simultaneously introducing the spike protein of SHC014 into the backbone of MA15 CoV and adding in five nucleotide Gain-of-Function substitutions, Zhengli and Baric were working to make Gain-of-Function changes in the spike protein of HKU4, also known as Tylonycteris bat coronavirus HKU4.[57] As already discussed, HKU4 does not infect human cells. By the end of this research, Baric and Zhengli had taken a virus that could not infect human cells and turned it into a virus that could and did:

> To evaluate the potential genetic changes required for HKU4 to infect human cells, **we reengineered** HKU4 spike, aiming to build its capacity to mediate viral entry into human cells. To this end, **we introduced two single mutations**, S746R and N762A, into HKU4 spike. . . . Moreover, mutations in these motifs in coronavirus spikes have **demonstrated dramatic effects on viral entry into human cells**.

Baric and Zhengli continued:

> HKU4 pseudoviruses bearing either the **reengineered** hPPC motif or the **reengineered** hECP motif were **able to enter human cells**, whereas HKU4 pseudoviruses bearing both of the reengineered human protease motifs entered human cells. . . . The two mutations adaptive to human cellular proteases **transformed MERS-CoV spike from completely lacking to fully possessing the capacity to mediate viral entry into human cells**.[58] [Emphasis added.]

This Gain-of-Function research turning a noninfectious coronavirus into an infective one and was paid for by NIH Grants RO1AI089728 and RO1AI110700.

Despite this evidence and the money funneled to Peter Daszak at EcoHealth Alliance, Peter Daszak led an intentional and knowing effort, along with other scientists, to divert attention from the lab origins of SARS-CoV-2 and Gain-of-Function research. This effort went so far as to recruit other scientists in the world to join with him in March 2020[59] to denounce a laboratory origin—insisting that the scientific community support Daszak and others in a zoonotic[60] origin of this bioweapon. Daszak concluded their "statement" by stating, "We declare no competing interests."

When the World Health Organization (WHO) sent a team of "experts" to the Wuhan Institute of Virology (WIV) in January 2021, Peter Daszak, who was the only American on the team and headed it, convinced the remainder of the team that the missing WIV data was "irrelevant."[61]

In an effort to demonstrate my disapproval and to protest the ever-deteriorating objectivity of our scientific journals, I resigned from *Lancet* as an external clinical reviewer in 2020 after almost two decades.

One cannot help but be struck by the significant amount of information in the published literature showing the source of funding for these Gain-of-Function research projects and those involved in conducting the experiments. One also cannot remain incognizant of the Gain-of-Function research carried out on the spike protein of coronaviruses and SARS-CoV-2 and the efforts to retroactively attempt to cover the source of that funding.[62]

BIOTECHNOLOGY, HEALTH, NEWS   DECEMBER 16, 2020

Peter Daszak's EcoHealth Alliance Has Hidden Almost $40 Million In Pentagon Funding And Militarized Pandemic Science

by Sam Husseini

"Pandemics are like terrorist attacks: We know roughly where they originate and what's responsible for them, but we don't know exactly when the next one will happen. They need to be handled the same way — by identifying all possible sources and dismantling those before the next pandemic strikes."

This statement was written in the *New York Times* earlier this year by Peter Daszak. Daszak is the longtime president of the EcoHealth Alliance ☒, a New York-based non-profit whose claimed focus is pandemic prevention. But the EcoHealth Alliance, it turns out, is at the very centre of the COVID-19 pandemic in many ways.

To depict the pandemic in such militarized terms is, for Daszak, a commonplace. In an Oct. 7 online talk organized by Columbia University's School of International and Public Affairs ☒, Daszak presented a slide titled "Donald Rumsfeld's Prescient Speech.":

"There are known knowns; there are things we know that we know. There are known unknowns; that is to say, there are things that we know we don't know. But there are also unknown unknowns — there are things we don't know we don't know." (This Rumsfeld quote is in fact from a news conference)

CHAPTER 3

The Paper Trail of the US Funding for Gain-of-Function Research

In President Dwight D. Eisenhower's farewell speech to the nation, he warned of a great threat to the United States posed by the military-industrial complex:

> In the councils of government we must guard against the acquisition of unwarranted influence . . . by the military-industrial complex. The potential for the disastrous rise of misplaced power exists and will persist.
>
> We must never let the weight of this combination endanger our liberties or democratic processes. We should take *nothing* for granted.
>
> We must be alert to the equal and opposite danger that public policy could, itself, become the captive of a scientific-technological elite.[1]

If you do not think the United States federal government has a track record of conducting unauthorized, nonconsenting research upon its citizens and military, then you have not been looking at the record. It has a record of atrocities[2] and of hiding the truth.[3]

By October 2014 the US government had issued a policy statement regarding Gain-of-Function research, including the following restrictions:

> "New [US government] funding will not be released for gain-of-function research projects that may be reasonably anticipated to confer attributes to influenza, MERS, or SARS viruses such that the virus would have enhanced

pathogenicity and/or transmissibility in mammals via the respiratory route. The research funding pause would not apply to characterization or testing of naturally occurring influenza, MERS, and SARS viruses, unless the tests are reasonably anticipated to increase transmissibility and/or pathogenicity.[4]

However, in a footnote to the policy statement, the federal government also decided that this moratorium on Gain-of-Function did *not* apply if the federal government considered the research was "urgent" for "public health or national security."[5] That's an interesting statement, given the Department of Defense (DoD) was funding Gain-of-Funding research—including providing funding and a policy advisor to Peter Daszak at EcoHealth:

> An exception from the research pause may be obtained if the head of the USG [US government] funding agency determines that the research is urgently necessary to protect the public health or national security.

In the previous chapter, we looked at some of the published Gain-of-Function research carried out by Ralph S. Baric and Shi Zhengli-Li. In those papers, we were able to put together the publication paper trail showing how these and other researchers affiliated with Baric, Zhengli, and Peter Daszak of EcoHealth meticulously worked on changing coronaviruses to make them more infective and harmful to humans.

These and other researchers received funding from a variety of US federal agencies, including the Department of Defense, Health and Human Services, National Science Foundation, US Agency for International Development, Homeland Security, Department of Commerce, Department of Agriculture, and Department of the Interior, in addition to receiving funding from the Helmsley, Rockefeller, and Gates Foundations—all intertwined with Jeffrey Epstein, as seen in the published papers and grants shown in this book.

In this chapter, we are going to lay to rest any question regarding the funding of these individuals for Gain-of-Function research by the US federal government. What follows is some of that money trail beginning with a report published on the UCLA Department of Epidemiology School of Public Health website in February 2002, entitled *War on Health*:

> **Diseases** arising from camp life, social disruption and unhygienic field hospitals **have killed far more soldiers than has battle**.
>   That is the cheerful implication of the otherwise ominous fact that President Bush's **budget** asks Congress to more than **quadruple**

spending—from $1.4 billion to $5.9 billion—on **bioterrorism**. Last week Defense Secretary Donald **Rumsfeld** was unspecific in saying "it is likely" terrorist attacks "will grow vastly more deadly" than those of Sept. 11. But **budgets** often make **government's thinking clear**, and the **bioterrorism money** may imply Rumsfeld's meaning.

Dr. Anthony **Fauci**, director of the National Institute of Allergy and Infectious Diseases at the National Institutes of Health, says this infusion of **money** will **accelerate** our understanding of the biology and pathogenesis of microbes **that can be used in attacks**, and the biology of the microbes' hosts—human beings and their immune systems. One result should be more effective **vaccines** with less toxicity. [Emphasis added.][6]

From this report, it is clear that the US federal government, including Donald Rumsfeld and Anthony Fauci, have decided to spend massive amounts of money on bioterrorism:

SOME OF THE MONEY FROM THE DEPARTMENT OF DEFENSE (DOD)[7]

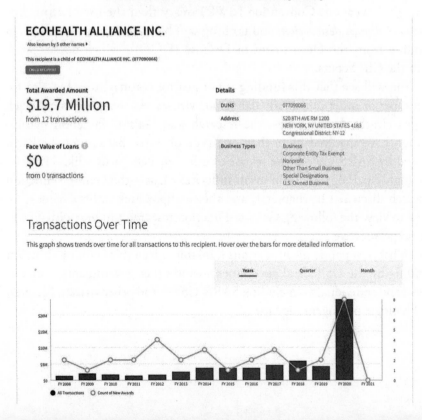

As you look through the following information you will notice that EcoHealth received more than the $19.7 million shown in the previous graphic. This represents only half of the $38,949,941 it actually received from the Department of Defense. The funding goes way beyond merely working on Gain-of-Function for SARS-CoV-2. This funding pays for work on a number of other viruses, raising serious concerns about new pandemics resulting from Gain-of-Function research.

As you look through most of these documents, the source and purpose of the funding, the award identification number, and the amount, you will notice a frequent recurring type of program funding—*weapons of mass destruction.*

CFDA Program / Assistance Listing ⓘ

12.351 - SCIENTIFIC RESEARCH - COMBATING
WEAPONS OF MASS DESTRUCTION
VIEW MORE INFO ABOUT THIS PROGRAM

Nothing speaks more clearly about this research and violation of the Biological Weapons Convention (BWC) treaty than the use of terms like *weapons of mass destruction,* and nothing says biological weapon more than funding from the Department of Defense (DOD)—which doesn't work with the Girl Scouts.

You will see that this funding is not just for coronaviruses but also for a number of other potentially dangerous viruses. As the government track record clearly demonstrates, the research and Gain-of-Function manipulation have involved more than one type of virus. Because of the harm caused by SARS-CoV-2, the release of other virulent viruses like H5N1— the highly pathogenic Asian avian influenza virus—the Gain-of-Function research discussed in chapter 1, and the smallpox and anthrax fiascos, we need to view the following Gain-of-Function research funding with a newfound perspective.

What new pandemic now awaits humanity given this Gain-of-Function funding by the US federal government—and other governments, corporations, and individuals—including SARS-CoV-2 and other viruses, bacteria, and biologic pathogenic agents?

Defense Threat Reduction Agency (DOD)

2015 Award ID HDTRA115C0041 for the amount of $2,217,037.00
2016 Award ID HDTRA115C0041 for the amount of $2,262,641.00[8]

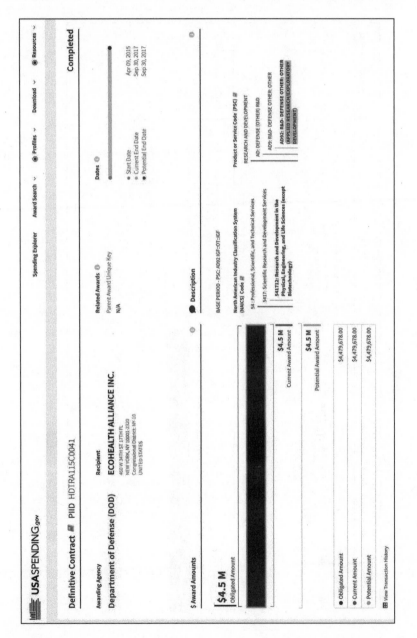

Defense Threat Reduction Agency (DOD)

2017 Award ID HDTRA11710037 for the amount of $721,249.00
2018 Award ID HDTRA11710037 for the amount of $883,274.00 [9, 10, 11, 12]

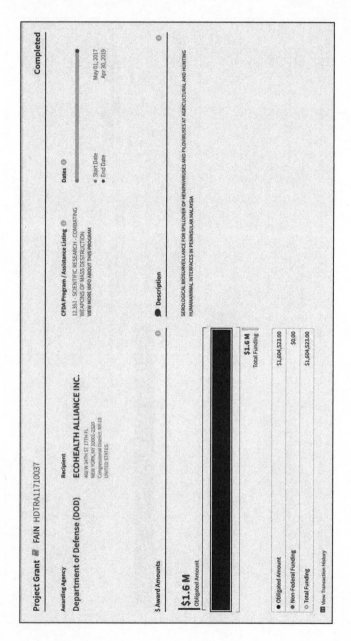

Home   Search   Data Bank   Data Services   Help

SAM.GOV (beta)

☷ Follow

ASSISTANCE LISTINGS

Scientific Research - Combating Weapons of Mass Destruction

⚠ Note: This Assistance Listing was not updated by the issuing agency in 2021. Please contact the issuing agency listed under "Contact Information" for more information.

Assistance Listing
Overview
Authorizations
Financial Information
Criteria for Applying
Applying for Assistance
Compliance Requirements
Contact Information
History

Sub-tier
DEFENSE THREAT REDUCTION AGENCY (DTRA)

CFDA Number
12.351

Related Federal Assistance
Not Applicable.

View available opportunities on Grants.gov related to this Assistance Listing ☍

Overview

Objectives

To support and stimulate basic, applied and advanced research at educational or research institutions, non-profit organizations, and commercial firms, which support the advancement of fundamental knowledge and understanding of the sciences with an emphasis on exploring new and innovative research for combating or countering Weapons of Mass Destruction (WMD).

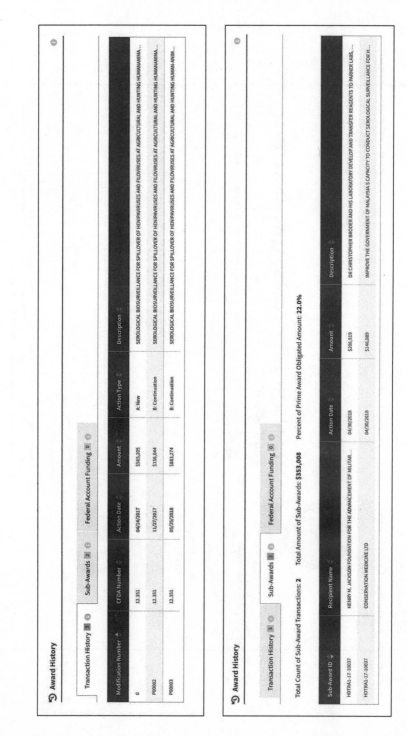

Defense Threat Reduction Agency (DOD)

2019 Award ID HDTRA11910033 for the amount of $998,437.00
2020 Award ID HDTRA11910033 for the amount of $3,990,550.00 [13, 14]

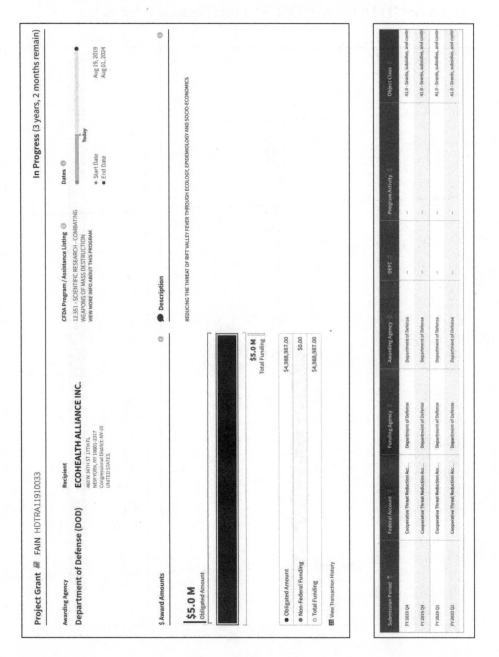

Defense Threat Reduction Agency (DOD)

2013 Award ID HDTRA113C0029 for the amount of $1,371,611.00
2014 Award ID HDTRA113C0029 for the amount of $957,145.00
2015 Award ID HDTRA113C0029 for the amount of $-103,622.00 [15, 16]

Department of Defense (DOD)

2014 Award ID HDTRA11410029 (#1) for the amount of $992,699.00
2015 Award ID HDTRA11410029 (#1) for the amount of $978,784.00
2016 Award ID HDTRA11410029 (#1) for the amount of $970,536.00 [17, 18]

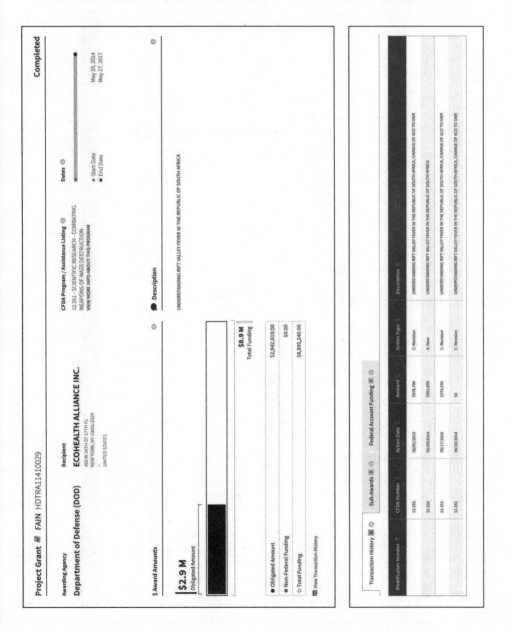

Defense Threat Reduction Agency (DOD)

2017 Award ID HDTRA11410029 (#2) for the amount of $996,147.00
2018 Award ID HDTRA11410029 (#2) for the amount of $998,193.00 [19, 20]

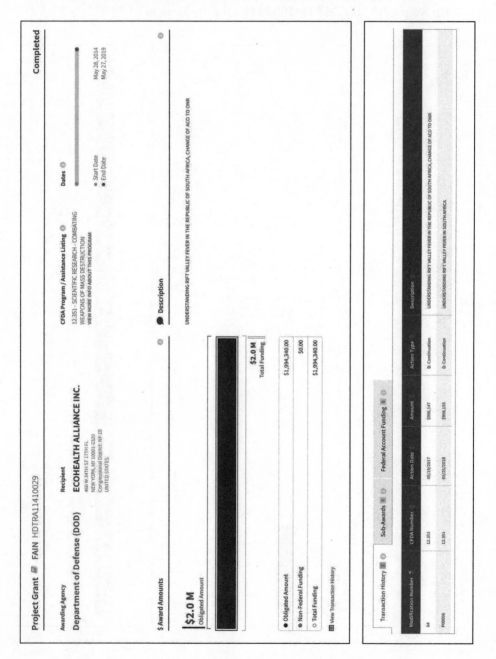

Defense Threat Reduction Agency (DOD)

2020 Award ID HDTRA12010016 for the amount of $4,912,818.00 [21, 22]

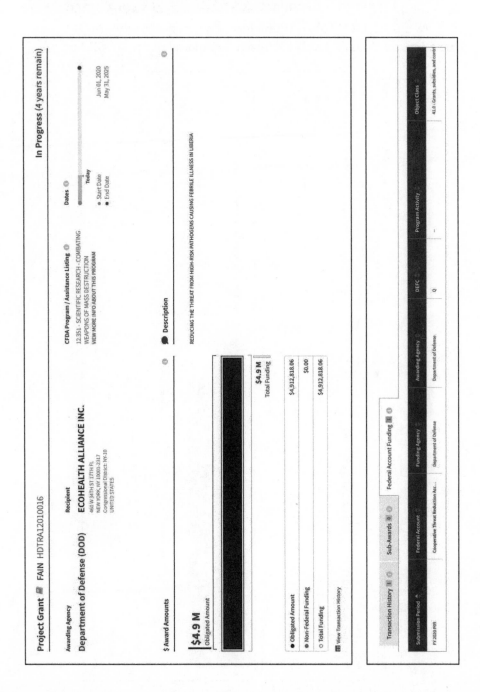

Defense Threat Reduction Agency (DOD)
2017 Award ID HDTRA11710064 for the amount of $782,330.00
2018 Award ID HDTRA11710064 for the amount of $2,203,917.00
2019 Award ID HDTRA11710064 for the amount of $1,995,247.00
2020 Award ID HDTRA11710064 for the amount of $1,509,531.00 [23, 24, 25]

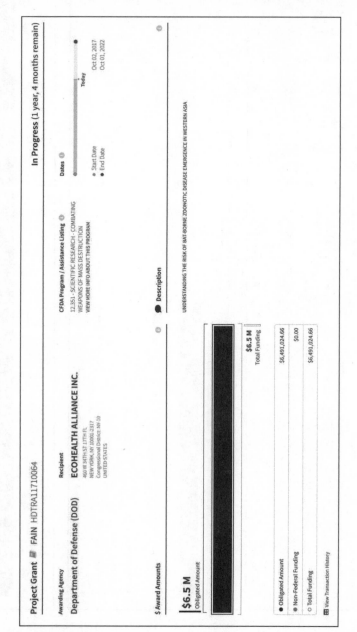

Transaction History | **Sub-Awards** | **Federal Account Funding**

Modification Number	CFDA Number	Action Date	Amount	Action Type	Description
0	12.351	09/05/2017	$782,330	A: New	UNDERSTANDING THE RISK OF BAT-BORNE ZOONOTIC DISEASE EMERGENCE IN WESTERN ASIA
P00001	12.351	05/25/2018	$1,101,959	B: Continuation'	UNDERSTANDING THE RISK OF BAT-BORNE ZOONOTIC DISEASE EMERGENCE IN WESTERN ASIA
P00001	12.351	05/25/2018	$1,101,058	B: Continuation	UNDERSTANDING THE RISK OF BAT-BORNE ZOONOTIC DISEASE EMERGENCE IN WESTERN ASIA
P00002	12.351	05/22/2019	$997,624	B: Continuation	UNDERSTANDING THE RISK OF BAT-BORN ZOONOTIC DISEASE EMERGENCE IN WESTERN ASIA
P00002	12.351	05/01/2019	$997,623	B: Continuation	UNDERSTANDING THE RISK OF BAT-BORN ZOONOTIC DISEASE EMERGENCE IN WESTERN ASIA
P00003	12.351	03/23/2020	$1,509,531	B: Continuation	UNDERSTANDING THE RISK OF BAT-BORNE ZOONOTIC DISEASE EMERGENCE IN WESTERN ASIA

Transaction History | **Sub-Awards** | **Federal Account Funding**

Submission Period	Federal Account	Funding Agency	Awarding Agency	DEFC	Program Activity	Object Class
FY 2019 Q3	Cooperative Threat Reduction Acc...	Department of Defense	Department of Defense	-	-	41.0 - Grants, subsidies, and contr...
FY 2020 Q2	Cooperative Threat Reduction Acc...	Department of Defense	Department of Defense	-	-	41.0 - Grants, subsidies, and contr...

Defense Threat Reduction Agency (DOD)

2020 Award ID HDTRA12010018 for the amount of $4,995,106.00 [26, 27]

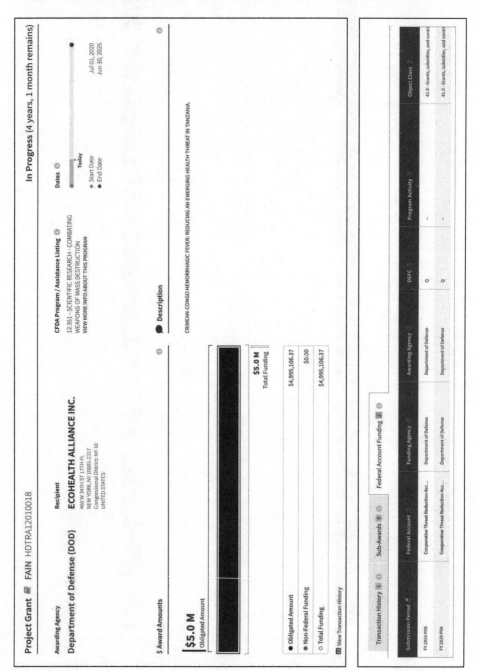

Uniformed Services University of the Health Sciences (DOD)
2020 Award ID HU00012010031 for the amount of $1,360,002.00 [28, 29]

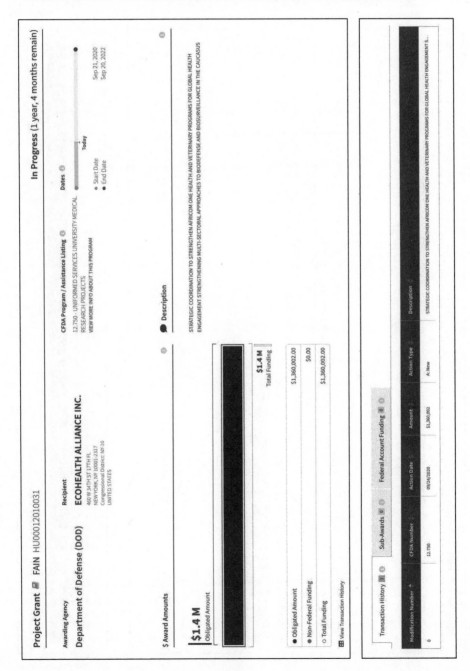

Defense Threat Reduction Agency (DOD)

2020 Award ID HDTRA12010029 for the amount of $2,956,309.00 [30, 31]

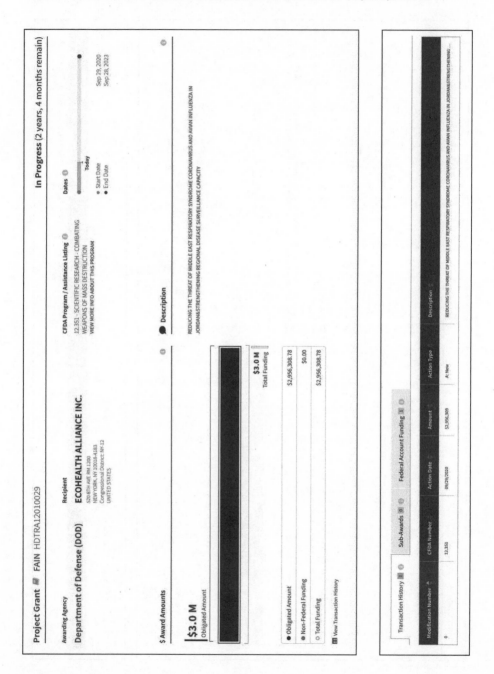

Above and beyond money to pay for research, the Department of Defense provided Peter Daszak of EcoHealth one more important resource: a policy advisor by the name of David Franz. Colonel Franz is a former deputy commander for Fort Detrick.

Fort Detrick, once known as the US biological weapons program center, is now known by the less threatening US Army Medical Research and Development Command (USAMRDC) and its biodefense agency, the US Army Medical Research Institute for Infectious Diseases (USAMRIID).[32] Dr. Franz serves on the Boards of the Federation of American Scientists and Integrated Nano-Technologies, LLC. His bio on the Kansas State University website states the following:

> Dr. Franz was the chief inspector on three United Nations Special Commission biological warfare inspection missions to Iraq and served as technical advisor on long-term monitoring. He also served as a member of the US-UK teams that visited Russia in support of the Trilateral Joint Statement on Biological Weapons and as a member of the Trilateral Experts' Committee for biological weapons negotiations. He was **technical editor** for the "**Textbook of Military Medicine on Medical Aspects of Chemical and Biological Warfare**" released in 1997. Current standing committee appointments include the National Academy of Sciences Committee on International Security and Arms Control where he **chairs the "biological panel**," American Society for Microbiology Committee on **Biodefense** of the Public and Scientific Affairs Board, and the Senior Technical Advisory Committee of the National **Biodefense** Countermeasures Analysis Center (DHS). He serves as a senior mentor to the Program for Emerging Leaders at the National Defense University. He also serves on the boards of the Elizabeth R. Griffin Research Foundation and Integrated Nano-Technologies LLC. Dr. Franz holds an adjunct appointment as professor for the Department of Diagnostic Medicine and Pathobiology at the College of Veterinary Medicine, Kansas State University. The current focus of his activities relates to the role of international engagement in public health and the life sciences as a component of **global biosecurity policy**. Domestically, he continues to encourage thoughtfulness when regulating research in the name of security, thereby minimizing negative impact on progress in the life sciences. [Emphasis added.][33]

SOME OF THE MONEY FROM HEALTH
AND HUMAN SERVICES (HHS)

National Institutes of Health—NIH (HHS)

2008 Award ID RO1TW005869 for the amount of $697,356.00

2009 Award ID RO1TW005869 for the amount of $1,001,985.00

2010 Award ID RO1TW005869 for the amount of $763,008.00

2011 Award ID RO1TW005869 for the amount of $761,374.00

2012 Award ID RO1TW005869 for the amount of $501,437.00 [34, 35, 36]

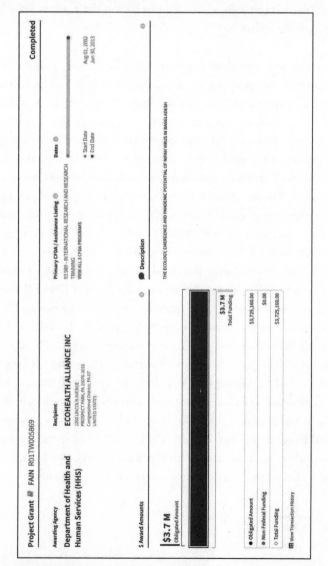

Transaction History | **Sub-Awards** | **Federal Account Funding**

Modification Number	CFDA Number	Action Date	Amount	Action Type	Description
000	93.989	06/14/2012	$6,962	B: Continuation	THE ECOLOGY, EMERGENCE AND PANDEMIC POTENTIAL OF NIPAH VIRUS IN BANGLADESH
000	93.989	09/07/2008	$502,356	B: Continuation	THE ECOLOGY, EMERGENCE AND PANDEMIC POTENTIAL OF NIPAH VIRUS IN BANGLADESH
001	93.989	08/28/2011	$494,455	B: Continuation	THE ECOLOGY, EMERGENCE AND PANDEMIC POTENTIAL OF NIPAH VIRUS IN BANGLADESH
001	93.989	09/26/2008	$150,000	B: Continuation	THE ECOLOGY, EMERGENCE AND PANDEMIC POTENTIAL OF NIPAH VIRUS IN BANGLADESH
001	93.989	08/06/2010	$499,998	B: Continuation	THE ECOLOGY, EMERGENCE AND PANDEMIC POTENTIAL OF NIPAH VIRUS IN BANGLADESH
001	93.989	08/27/2009	$499,975	B: Continuation	THE ECOLOGY, EMERGENCE AND PANDEMIC POTENTIAL OF NIPAH VIRUS IN BANGLADESH
001	93.989	07/27/2012	$494,455	B: Continuation	THE ECOLOGY, EMERGENCE AND PANDEMIC POTENTIAL OF NIPAH VIRUS IN BANGLADESH
002	93.999	09/10/2010	$63,018	B: Continuation	THE ECOLOGY, EMERGENCE AND PANDEMIC POTENTIAL OF NIPAH VIRUS IN BANGLADESH
002	93.999	09/29/2011	$266,919	B: Continuation	THE ECOLOGY, EMERGENCE AND PANDEMIC POTENTIAL OF NIPAH VIRUS IN BANGLADESH
002	93.989	09/26/2008	$45,000	B: Continuation	THE ECOLOGY, EMERGENCE AND PANDEMIC POTENTIAL OF NIPAH VIRUS IN BANGLADESH

Transaction History | **Sub-Awards** | **Federal Account Funding**

Modification Number	CFDA Number	Action Date	Amount	Action Type	Description
001	93.989	08/27/2009	$499,975	B: Continuation	THE ECOLOGY, EMERGENCE AND PANDEMIC POTENTIAL OF NIPAH VIRUS IN BANGLADESH
001	93.989	07/27/2012	$494,455	B: Continuation	THE ECOLOGY, EMERGENCE AND PANDEMIC POTENTIAL OF NIPAH VIRUS IN BANGLADESH
002	93.999	09/10/2010	$63,018	B: Continuation	THE ECOLOGY, EMERGENCE AND PANDEMIC POTENTIAL OF NIPAH VIRUS IN BANGLADESH
002	93.999	09/26/2011	$266,919	B: Continuation	THE ECOLOGY, EMERGENCE AND PANDEMIC POTENTIAL OF NIPAH VIRUS IN BANGLADESH
002	93.989	09/26/2008	$45,000	B: Continuation	THE ECOLOGY, EMERGENCE AND PANDEMIC POTENTIAL OF NIPAH VIRUS IN BANGLADESH
003	93.701	09/01/2009	$204,688	B: Continuation	THE ECOLOGY, EMERGENCE AND PANDEMIC POTENTIAL OF NIPAH VIRUS IN BANGLADESH
003	93.999	09/13/2010	$199,992	B: Continuation	THE ECOLOGY, EMERGENCE AND PANDEMIC POTENTIAL OF NIPAH VIRUS IN BANGLADESH
004	93.701	09/02/2009	$51,225	B: Continuation	THE ECOLOGY, EMERGENCE AND PANDEMIC POTENTIAL OF NIPAH VIRUS IN BANGLADESH
005	93.989	09/21/2009	$199,698	B: Continuation	THE ECOLOGY, EMERGENCE AND PANDEMIC POTENTIAL OF NIPAH VIRUS IN BANGLADESH
006	93.989	09/22/2009	$46,399	B: Continuation	THE ECOLOGY, EMERGENCE AND PANDEMIC POTENTIAL OF NIPAH VIRUS IN BANGLADESH

National Institutes of Health—NIH (HHS)
2007 Award ID K08AI067549 for the amount of $130,950.00
2009 Award ID K08AI067549 for the amount of $180,944.00
2010 Award ID K08AI067549 for the amount of $130,950.00[37, 38]

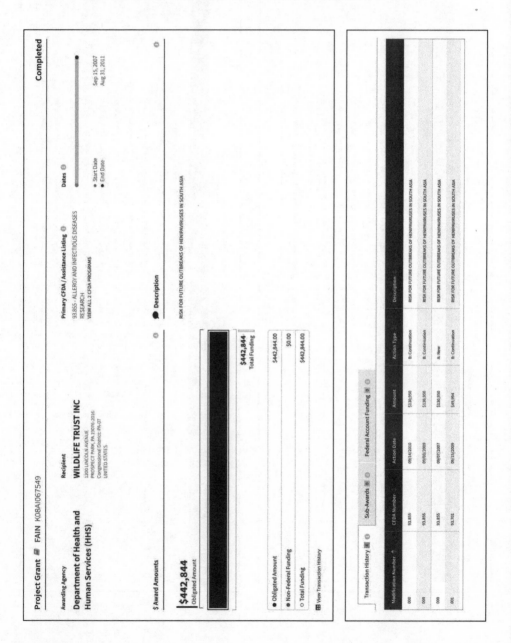

National Institutes of Health—NIH (HHS)

2007 Award ID R56TW009502 for the amount of $300,000.00[39, 40]

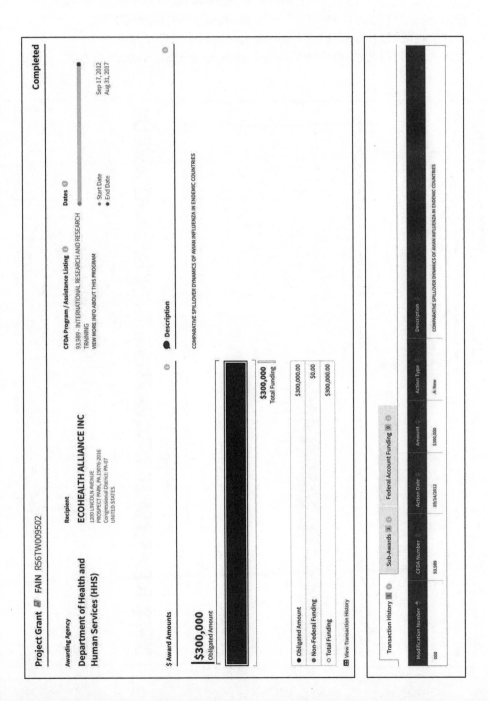

National Institute of Allergy and Infectious Diseases (HHS-NIH)

2014 Award ID R01AI110964 for the amount of $666,442.00
2015 Award ID R01AI110964 for the amount of $630,445.00
2016 Award ID R01AI110964 for the amount of $611,090.00
2017 Award ID R01AI110964 for the amount of $597,112.00
2018 Award ID R01AI110964 for the amount of $581,646.00[41, 42, 43, 44]

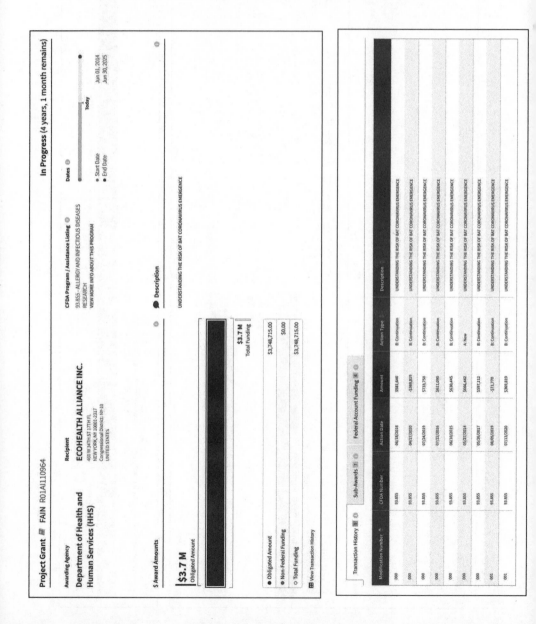

Transaction History | Sub-Awards | Federal Account Funding

Total Count of Sub-Award Transactions: 7   Total Amount of Sub-Awards: $799,717   Percent of Prime Award Obligated Amount: 21.3%

Sub-Award ID	Recipient Name	Action Date	Amount	Description
1R01AI110964-01	WUHAN INSTITUTE OF VIROLOGY CHINESE ACADEMY OF SCIENCES CAP...	05/31/2019	$66,500	CONDUCT HIGH-QUALITY TESTING, SEQUENCING, AND ANALYSES OF FIELD SAMPLES; MAINTENANCE OF C...
1R01AI110964-01	WUHAN INSTITUTE OF VIROLOGY CHINESE ACADEMY OF SCIENCES CAP...	05/31/2018	$133,000	CONDUCT HIGH-QUALITY TESTING, SEQUENCING, AND ANALYSES OF FIELD SAMPLES; MAINTENANCE OF C...
1R01AI110964-01	WUHAN INSTITUTE OF VIROLOGY CHINESE ACADEMY OF SCIENCES CAP...	05/31/2017	$133,000	CONDUCT HIGH-QUALITY TESTING, SEQUENCING, AND ANALYSES OF FIELD SAMPLES; MAINTENANCE OF C...
1R01AI110964-01	WUHAN INSTITUTE OF VIROLOGY CHINESE ACADEMY OF SCIENCES CAP...	05/31/2016	$133,000	CONDUCT HIGH-QUALITY TESTING, SEQUENCING, AND ANALYSIS OF FIELD SAMPLES; MAINTENANCE OF C...
1R01AI110964-01	WUHAN INSTITUTE OF VIROLOGY CHINESE ACADEMY OF SCIENCES CAP...	05/29/2015	$133,000	CONDUCT HIGH-QUALITY TESTING, SEQUENCING, AND ANALYSES OF FIELD SAMPLES; MAINTENANCE OF C...
1R01AI110964-01	WUHAN UNIVERSITY SCHOOL OF PUBLIC HEALTH	05/31/2017	$159,342	CONDUCT TARGETED SITE-ANALYSES, HUMAN BEHAVIORAL SURVEILLANCE INCLUDING QUALITATIVE AND ...
1R01AI110964-01	WUHAN UNIVERSITY SCHOOL OF PUBLIC HEALTH	05/31/2016	$41,875	CONDUCT TARGETED SITE-ANALYSES, HUMAN BEHAVIORAL SURVEILLANCE INCLUDING QUALITATIVE AND ...

Transaction History | Sub-Awards | Federal Account Funding

Submission Period	Federal Account	Funding Agency	Awarding Agency	DEFC	Program Activity	Object Class
FY 2017 Q3	National Institute of Allergy and Inf...	Department of Health and Human...	Department of Health and Human S...	-	:	41.0 - Grants, subsidies, and contri
FY 2018 Q3	National Institute of Allergy and Inf...	Department of Health and Human...	Department of Health and Human S...	-	:	41.0 - Grants, subsidies, and contri
FY 2019 Q4	National Institute of Allergy and Inf...	Department of Health and Human...	Department of Health and Human S...	-	:	41.0 - Grants, subsidies, and contri
FY 2019 Q4	National Institute of Allergy and Inf...	Department of Health and Human...	Department of Health and Human S...	-	:	41.0 - Grants, subsidies, and contri
FY 2020 P07	National Institute of Allergy and Inf...	Department of Health and Human...	Department of Health and Human S...	Q	:	41.0 - Grants, subsidies, and contri
FY 2020 P10	National Institute of Allergy and Inf...	Department of Health and Human...	Department of Health and Human S...	Q		41.0 - Grants, subsidies, and contri

CDC Office of Acquisition Services (HHS)

2011 Award ID HHSD2002011M41641P for the amount of $59,740.00
2013 Award ID HHSD2002011M41641P for the amount of $45,000.00
2016 Award ID HHSD2002011M41641P for the amount of $-5,446.00 [45, 46]

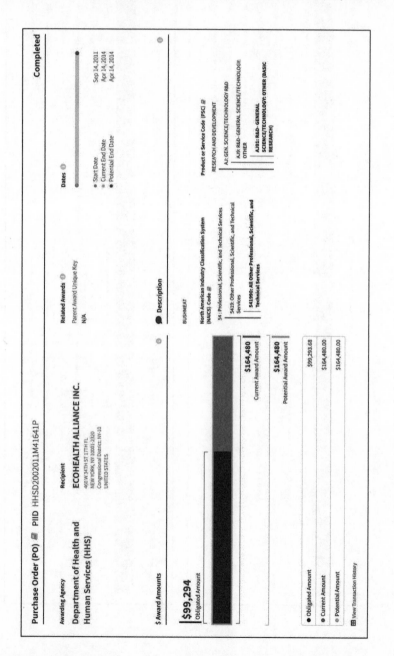

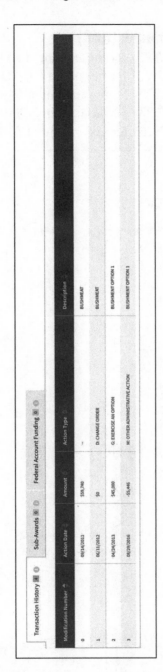

Notice that the description of this award is for *bushmeat*. Bushmeat comes from a variety of wild animals, including bats,[47] nonhuman primates (i.e., monkeys), rats, and antelope. It is illegal to bring this into the United States. (See appendix.)

National Institutes of Health (HHS)

2008 Award ID R01AI079231 for the amount of $534,989.00
2009 Award ID R01AI079231 for the amount of $535,156.00
2010 Award ID R01AI079231 for the amount of $480,423.00
2011 Award ID R01AI079231 for the amount of $510,005.00
2012 Award ID R01AI079231 for the amount of $518,980.00[48, 49]

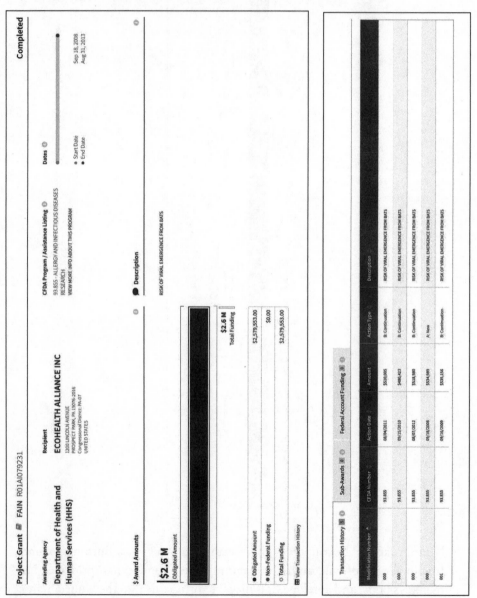

NIH National Institute of Allergy and Infectious Diseases (NIAID) (HHS)

2020 Award ID U01AI151797 for the amount of $1,546,744.00[50, 51, 52]

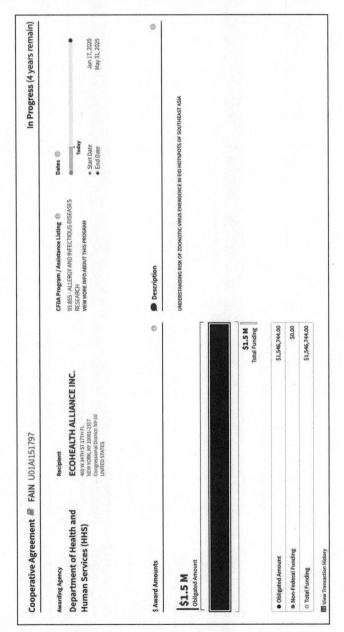

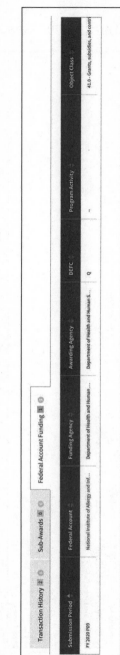

Transaction History 2 **Sub-Awards 0** **Federal Account Funding 1**

Modification Number	CFDA Number	Action Date	Amount	Action Type	Description
000	93.855	06/17/2020	$1,546,744	A: New	UNDERSTANDING RISK OF ZOONOTIC VIRUS EMERGENCE IN EID HOTSPOTS OF SOUTHEAST ASIA
001	93.855	06/28/2020	$0	A: New	UNDERSTANDING RISK OF ZOONOTIC VIRUS EMERGENCE IN EID HOTSPOTS OF SOUTHEAST ASIA

Transaction History 2 **Sub-Awards 0** **Federal Account Funding 1**

Submission Period	Federal Account	Funding Agency	Awarding Agency	DEFC	Program Activity	Object Class
FY 2020 P09	National Institute of Allergy and Inf…	Department of Health and Human …	Department of Health and Human S…	Q	-	41.0 - Grants, subsidies, and contri

Department of Health and Human Services (HHS)
2020 Award ID U01AI153420 for the amount of $580,858.00[53, 54, 55, 56]

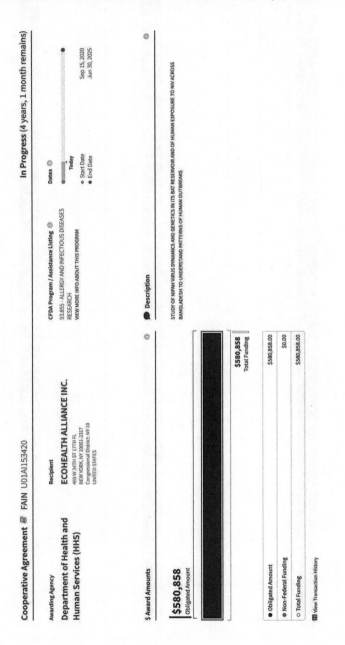

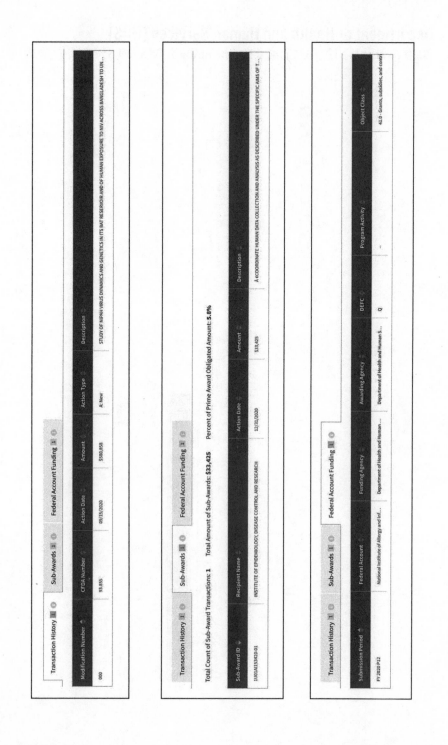

SOME OF THE MONEY FROM THE NATIONAL SCIENCE FOUNDATION (NSF)

National Science Foundation (NSF)

2016 Award ID 1618919 for the amount of $190,223.00

2017 Award ID 1618919 for the amount of $309,674.00[57, 58, 59]

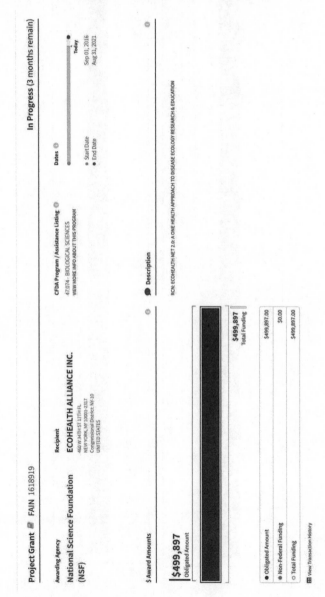

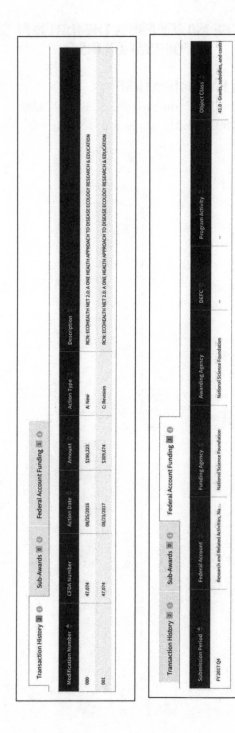

National Science Foundation (NSF)

2017 Award ID 1714394 for the amount of $138,000.00
2020 Award ID 1714394 for the amount of $-40,250.00[60]

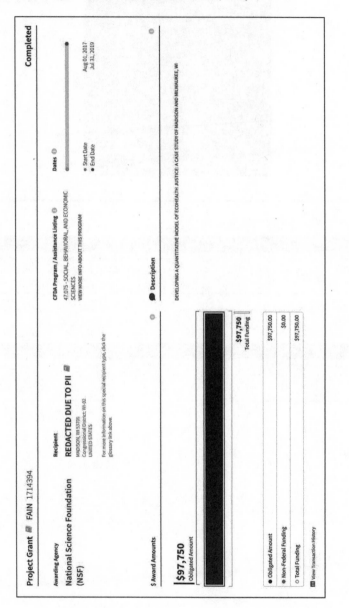

Note that information has been redacted on these documents.[61, 62, 63]

Redacted Due To PII

A recipient name of "REDACTED DUE TO PII" indicates that the associated financial assistance award was issued to an individual whose name and other Personally Identifiable Information (PII) were redacted, as required by law. Along with masking the individual's name with "REDACTED DUE TO PII," these records omit location information that would otherwise be present (street address and the last 4 digits of the ZIP code).

Transaction History	Sub-Awards	Federal Account Funding		

Modification Number	CFDA Number	Action Date	Amount	Action Type	Description
000	47.075	07/10/2017	$138,000	A: New	DEVELOPING A QUANTITATIVE MODEL OF ECOHEALTH JUSTICE: A CASE STUDY OF MADISON AND MILWAUKEE, WI
001	47.075	04/14/2020	-$40,250	C: Revision	DEVELOPING A QUANTITATIVE MODEL OF ECOHEALTH JUSTICE: A CASE STUDY OF MADISON AND MILWAUKEE, WI

Transaction History	Sub-Awards	Federal Account Funding		

Submission Period	Federal Account	Funding Agency	Awarding Agency	DEFC	Program Activity	Object Class
FY 2017 Q4	Research and Related Activities, Na...		National Science Foundation	--	--	41.0 - Grants, subsidies, and contri
FY 2020 P07	Research and Related Activities, Na...		National Science Foundation	Q	--	41.0 - Grants, subsidies, and contri

Division of Environmental Biology (NSF)

2010 Award ID 1015791 for the amount of $29,109.00
2012 Award ID 1015791 for the amount of $13,948.00
2013 Award ID 1015791 for the amount of $14,293.00
2014 Award ID 1015791 for the amount of $14,652.00[64, 65]

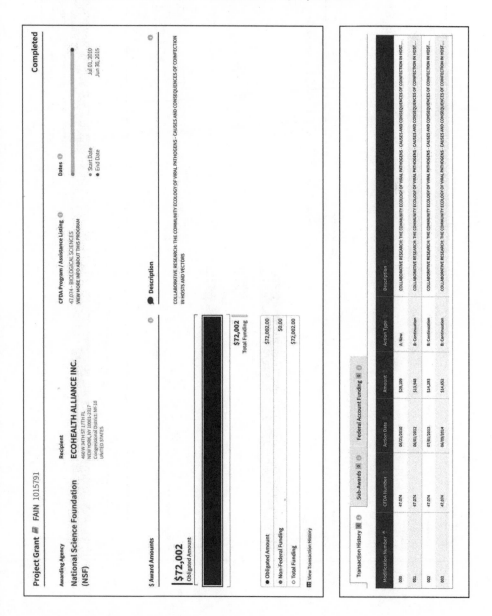

National Science Foundation (NSF)

2012 Award ID 1257513 for the amount of $22,890.00[66, 67]

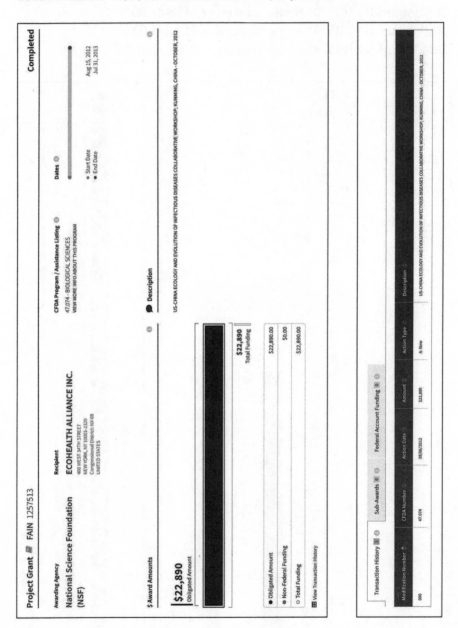

Division of Environmental Biology (NSF)

2010 Award ID 955897 for the amount of $99,611.00
2011 Award ID 955897 for the amount of $98,673.00
2012 Award ID 955897 for the amount of $99,919.00
2013 Award ID 955897 for the amount of $98,992.00
2014 Award ID 955897 for the amount of $99,926.00[68, 69]

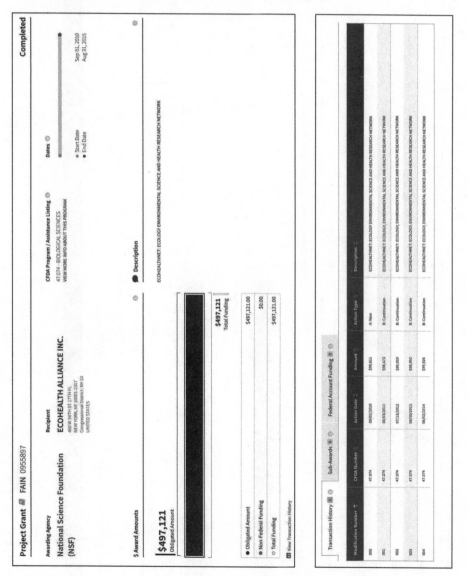

National Science Foundation (NSF)

2006 Award ID 0622391 for the amount of $503,291.00
2008 Award ID 0622391 for the amount of $428,794.00[70, 71]

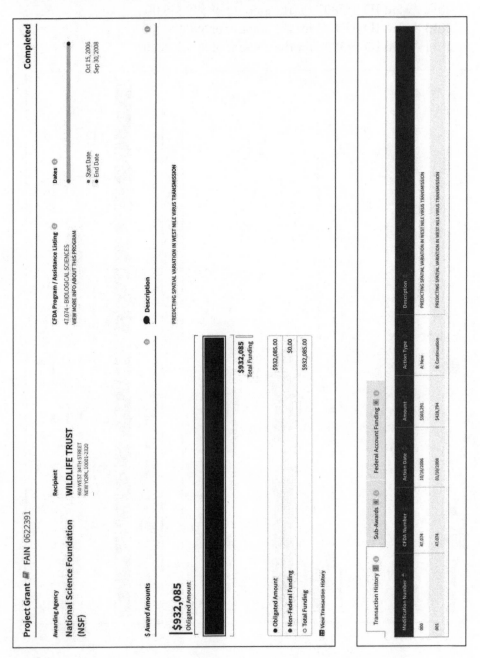

National Science Foundation (NSF)

2008 Award ID 0826779 for the amount of $468,673.00[72, 73]

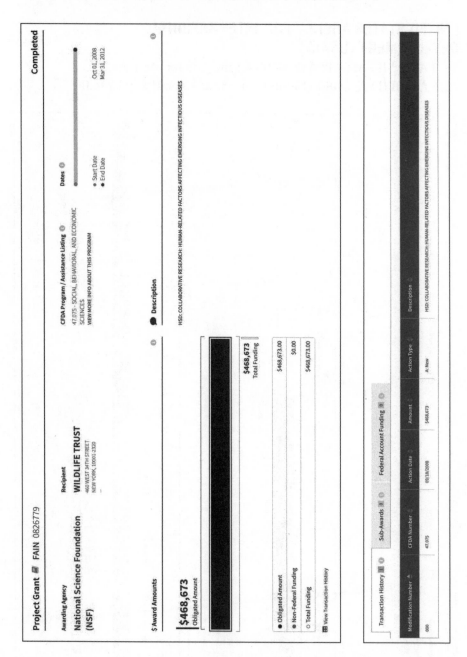

SOME OF THE MONEY FROM THE UNITED STATES AGENCY FOR INTERNATIONAL DEVELOPMENT (USAID)

UNITED STATES AGENCY FOR INTERNATIONAL DEVELOPMENT (USAID)

2013 Award ID AID486A1300005 for the amount of $1,999,203.00
2016 Award ID AID486A1300005 for the amount of $499,944.00[74, 75]

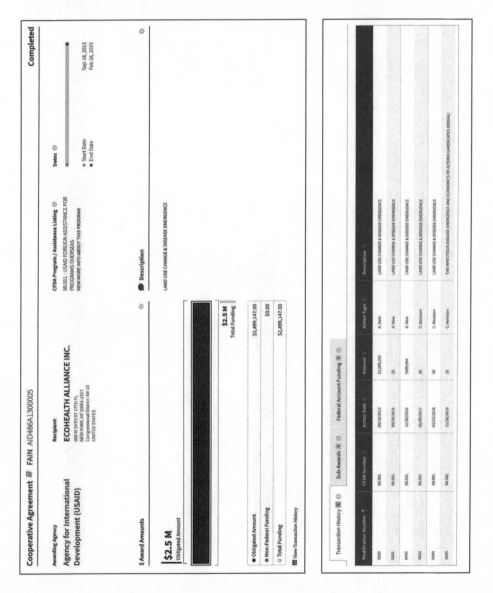

SOME OF THE MONEY FROM THE DEPARTMENT OF HOMELAND SECURITY (DHS)

Science and Technology Acquisition Division (DHS)

2019 Award ID 70RSAT19CB0000013 for the amount of $566,274.00[76, 77, 78]

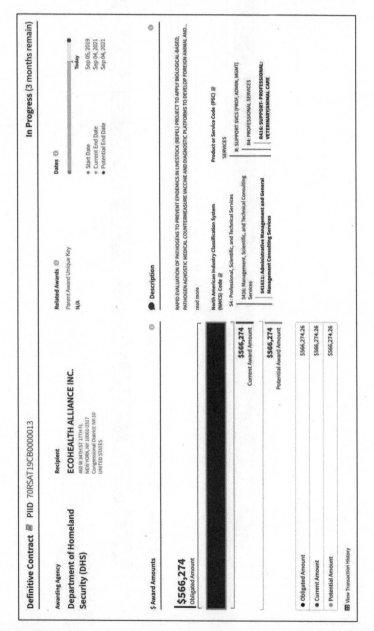

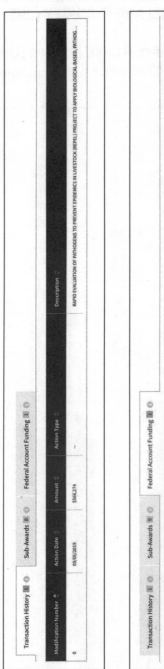

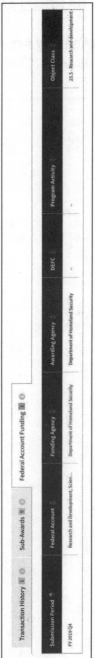

Office of Health Affairs Acquisition Division (DHS)

2016 Award ID HSHQDC16C00113 for the amount of $271,272.00
2017 Award ID HSHQDC16C00113 for the amount of $327,782.00
2018 Award ID HSHQDC16C00113 for the amount of $406,902.00[79, 80, 81]

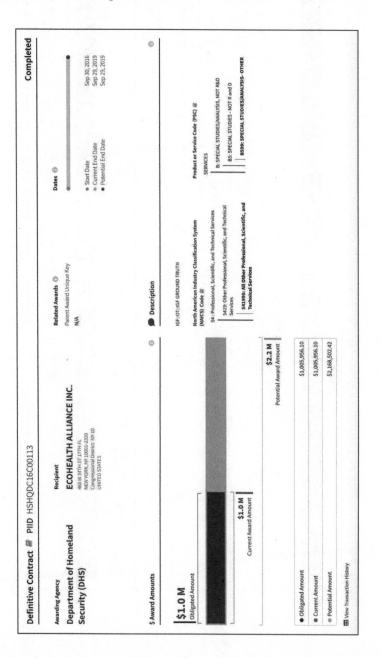

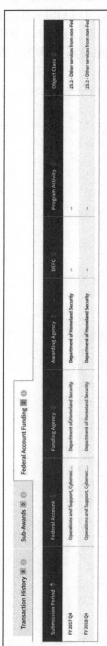

Transaction History | Sub-Awards | Federal Account Funding

Modification Number	Action Date	Amount	Action Type	Description
0	09/30/2016	$271,272	-	IGF::OT::IGF GROUND TRUTH
P00001	11/07/2016	$0	B: SUPPLEMENTAL AGREEMENT FOR WORK WITHIN SCOPE	IGF::OT::IGF GROUND TRUTH
P00002	01/03/2017	$0	M: OTHER ADMINISTRATIVE ACTION	IGF::OT::IGF COR CHANGE FOR THE ECOHEALTH ALLIANCE CONTRACT IN SUPPORT OF NBIC'S GROUNDTRUTH EFFORT
P00003	06/14/2017	$390,394	G: EXERCISE AN OPTION	IGF::OT::IGF COR CHANGE FOR THE ECOHEALTH ALLIANCE CONTRACT IN SUPPORT OF NBIC'S GROUNDTRUTH EFFORT
P00004	07/18/2017	-$67,112	M: OTHER ADMINISTRATIVE ACTION	IGF::OT::IGF ZERO DOLLAR PR TO REALLOCATE BASE CLIN FUNDING TO OPTION
P00005	08/28/2017	$4,500	C: FUNDING ONLY ACTION	IGF::OT::IGF ZERO DOLLAR PR TO REALLOCATE BASE CLIN FUNDING TO OPTION
P00006	04/20/2018	$0	M: OTHER ADMINISTRATIVE ACTION	IGF::OT::IGF THE PURPOSE OF THIS ZERO DOLLAR MODIFICATION IS TO CHANGE THE COR DUTIES FROM LCDR REAJUL MOJUMDER T...
P00007	09/11/2018	$406,902	G: EXERCISE AN OPTION	IGF::OT::IGF THE PURPOSE OF THIS ZERO DOLLAR MODIFICATION IS TO CHANGE THE COR DUTIES FROM LCDR REAJUL MOJUMDER T...

Transaction History | Sub-Awards | Federal Account Funding

Submission Period	Federal Account	Funding Agency	Awarding Agency	DEFC	Program Activity	Object Class
FY 2017 Q4	Operations and Support, Cybersec...	Department of Homeland Security	Department of Homeland Security	-	-	25.2 - Other services from non-Fed
FY 2018 Q4	Operations and Support, Cybersec...	Department of Homeland Security	Department of Homeland Security	-	-	25.2 - Other services from non-Fed

The National Biosurveillance Integration Center is involved in addressing weapons of mass destruction and countering weapons of mass destruction.[82] (See appendix.)[83]

This same agency works closely with the National LGBT Chamber of Commerce.[84]

Science and Technology Acquisition Division (DHS)

2017 Award ID 70RSAT18CB0031001 for the amount of $413,761.00

2018 Award ID 70RSAT18CB0031001 for the amount of $246,770.00

2019 Award ID 70RSAT18CB0031001 for the amount of $40,052.00[85, 86, 87]

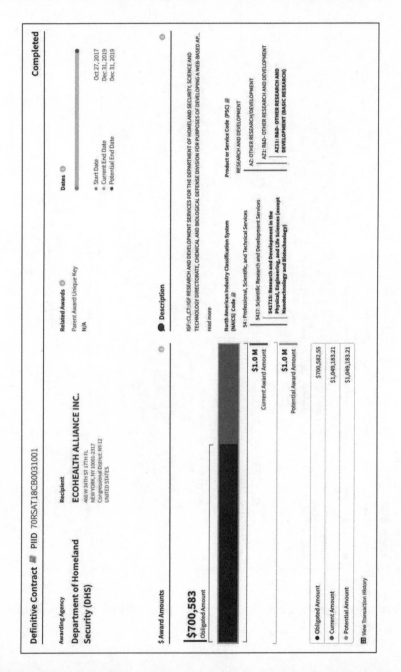

Transaction History 5 ⊕ | **Sub-Awards** 0 ⊕ | **Federal Account Funding** 3 ⊕

Modification Number	Action Date	Amount	Action Type	Description
0	10/27/2017	$413,761	-	IGF::CL::CT::IGF RESEARCH AND DEVELOPMENT SERVICES FOR THE DEPARTMENT OF HOMELAND SECURITY, SCIENCE AND TECHNOLO...
P00001	02/07/2018	$0	S: CHANGE PIID	IGF::CL::CT::IGF RESEARCH AND DEVELOPMENT SERVICES FOR THE DEPARTMENT OF HOMELAND SECURITY, SCIENCE AND TECHNOLO...
P00002	09/21/2018	$246,770	G: EXERCISE AN OPTION	IGF::CL::CT::IGF COMMIT FUNDING FOR INBOUND BIO-EVENT INFORMATION SYSTEM (IBIS)
P00003	08/01/2019	$40,052	C: FUNDING ONLY ACTION	ADDITIONAL FUNDING TO OPTION PERIOD 1, TASK 10 AND EXTEND PERIOD OF PERFORMANCE THROUGH DECEMBER 31, 2019.
P00004	01/21/2021	$0	K: CLOSE OUT	CLOSEOUT MODIFICATION

Transaction History 5 ⊕ | **Sub-Awards** 0 ⊕ | **Federal Account Funding** 3 ⊕

Submission Period	Federal Account	Funding Agency	Awarding Agency	DEFC	Program Activity	Object Class
FY 2018 Q3	Research and Development, Scien...	Department of Homeland Security	Department of Homeland Security	-	-	25.5 : Research and development ...
FY 2018 Q4	Research and Development, Scien...	Department of Homeland Security	Department of Homeland Security	-	-	25.5 : Research and development ...
FY 2019 Q4	Research and Development, Scien...	Department of Homeland Security	Department of Homeland Security	-	-	25.5 : Research and development ...

SOME OF THE MONEY FROM THE DEPARTMENT
OF COMMERCE (DOC)

Eastern Acquisition Division Kansas City (DOC)

2006 Award ID DOCWC133F06CN0251 for the amount of $256,120.00

2007 Award ID DOCWC133F06CN0251 for the amount of $263,228.00

2008 Award ID DOCWC133F06CN0251 for the amount of $276,685.00

2009 Award ID DOCWC133F06CN0251 for the amount of $220,700.00

2010 Award ID DOCWC133F06CN0251 for the amount of $225,200.00[88, 89]

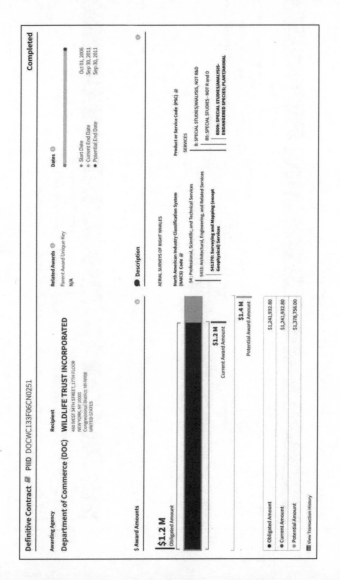

| Transaction History | Sub-Awards | Federal Account Funding |

Modification Number	Action Date	Amount	Action Type	Description
0	09/22/2006	$256,120	-	AERIAL SURVEYS OF RIGHT WHALES
1	09/06/2007	$263,228	G: EXERCISE AN OPTION	AERIAL SURVEYS OF RIGHT WHALES
2	02/08/2008	$0	D: CHANGE ORDER	AERIAL SURVEYS OF RIGHT WHALES
3	05/27/2008	$276,685	G: EXERCISE AN OPTION	AERIAL SURVEYS OF RIGHT WHALES
4	04/09/2009	$220,700	G: EXERCISE AN OPTION	OPTION YEAR 3
5	08/20/2010	$225,200	G: EXERCISE AN OPTION	OPTION YEAR 4
6	12/21/2010	$0	D: CHANGE ORDER	CHANGE IN KEY PERSONNEL
7	02/15/2011	$0	D: CHANGE ORDER	NAME CHANGE

SOME OF THE MONEY FROM THE US DEPARTMENT OF AGRICULTURE (USDA)

Department of Agriculture (USDA)

2008 Award ID 08-7100-0206-CA for the amount of $143,000.00[90, 91]

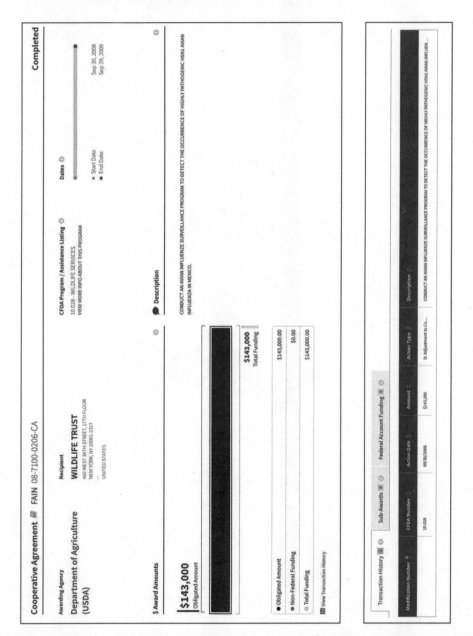

Department of Agriculture (USDA)
2009 Award ID 09-7100-0206-CA for the amount of $100,001.00[92, 93]

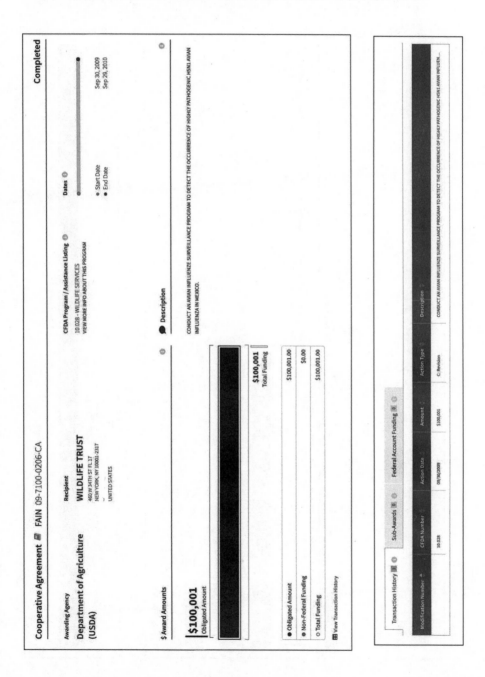

Animal and Plant Inspection Service (USDA)

2007 Award ID 07-7100-0237-CA for the amount of $403,700.00[94, 95]

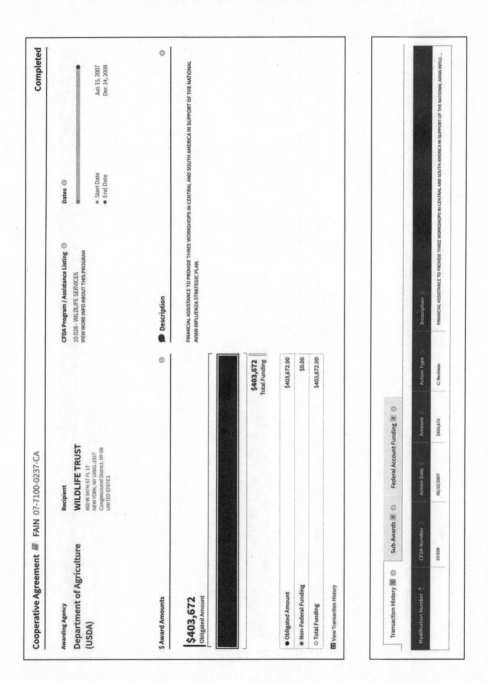

SOME OF THE MONEY FROM THE US DEPARTMENT OF THE INTERIOR (DOI)

Department of the Interior (DOI)

2012 Award ID F12AP01208 for the amount of $154,087.00[96, 97]

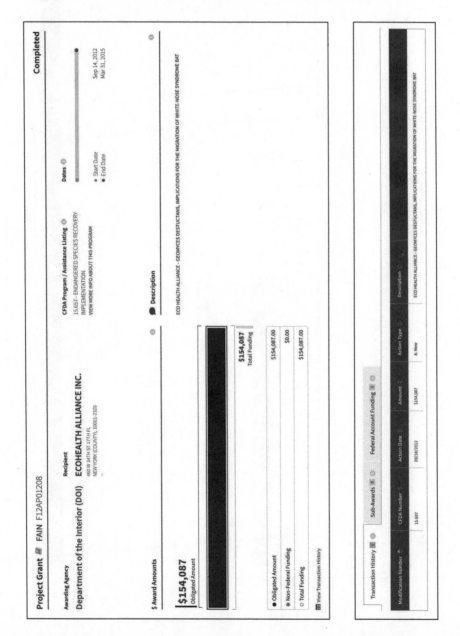

U.S. Fish & Wildlife Services (DOI)

2012 Award ID F12AP01117 for the amount of $44,499.00[98, 99]

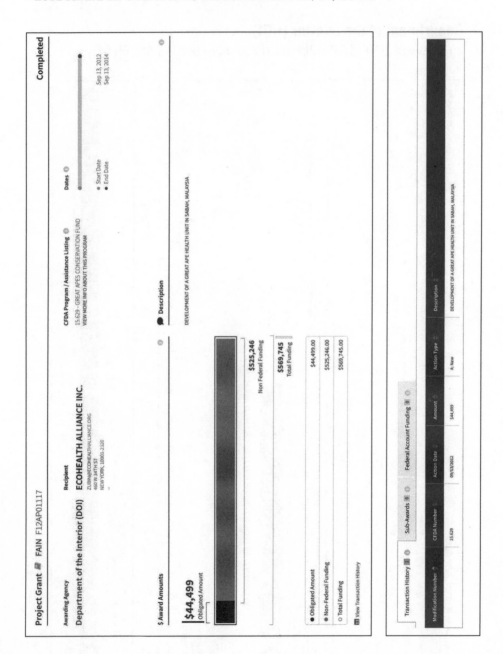

U.S. Fish & Wildlife Services (DOI)
2014 Award ID F14AP00269 for the amount of $29,988.00[100, 101]

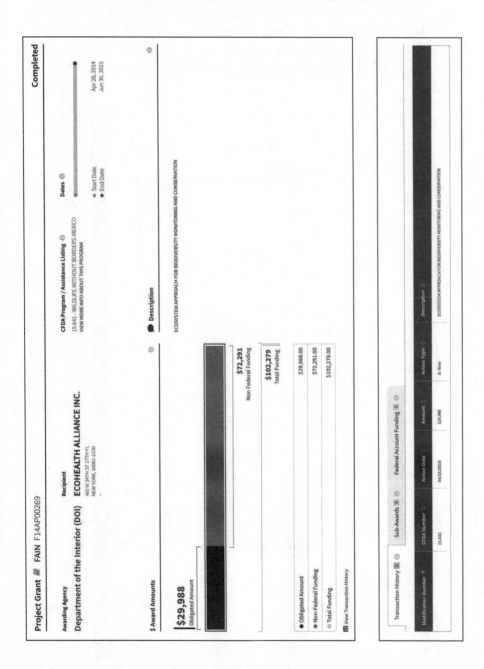

Office of Acquisition and Grants—Reston (DOI)
2004 Award ID ING04ERSA0526 for the amount of $16,000.00
2005 Award ID ING04ERSA0526 for the amount of $15,000.00
2006 Award ID ING04ERSA0526 for the amount of $10,000.00
2007 Award ID ING04ERSA0526 for the amount of $10,000.00
2008 Award ID ING04ERSA0526 for the amount of $10,000.00[102, 103]

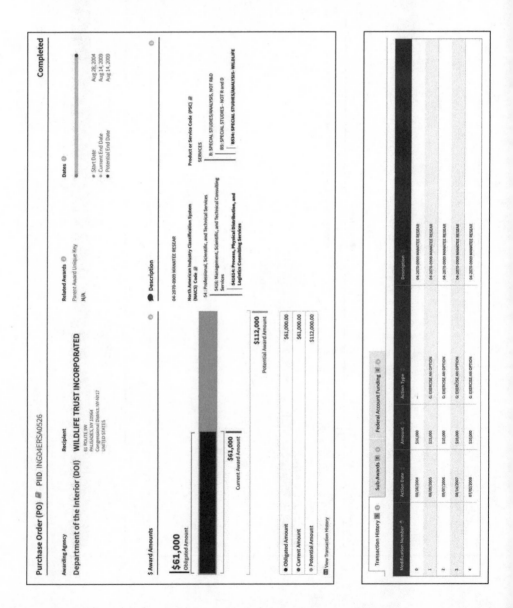

Department of the Interior (DOI)
2011 Award ID G05AC00002 for the amount of $-22,512.00[104, 105]

Project Grant FAIN G05AC00002

Completed

Awarding Agency
Department of the Interior (DOI)

Recipient
WILDLIFE TRUST INC.
460 WEST 34TH STREET, 17TH FLOOR
NEW YORK, 10001-2320
--

CFDA Program / Assistance Listing
15.808 - U.S. GEOLOGICAL SURVEY RESEARCH AND DATA COLLECTION
VIEW MORE INFO ABOUT THIS PROGRAM

Dates
- Start Date   Aug. 15, 2008
- End Date   Mar 01, 2009

$ Award Amounts

Chart Not Available
Data in this instance is not suitable for charting

Description

SEABIRD ECOLOGICAL ASSESSMENT NETWORK-SEANET

● Obligated Amount	-$22,512.00
● Non-Federal Funding	$0.00
○ Total Funding	-$22,512.00

View Transaction History

Transaction History   Sub-Awards   Federal Account Funding

Modification Number	CFDA Number	Action Date	Amount	Action Type	Description
0004	15.808	08/06/2011	-$22,512	A: New	SEABIRD ECOLOGICAL ASSESSMENT NETWORK-SEANET

The pattern of funding shows a flow from federal agencies aided and abetted by Dr. Anthony S. Fauci (since all of the grants were federal and Fauci was part of the group that reviewed GoF grants and other grants). This money eventually went to Peter Daszak of EcoHealth and then at least some of which went to Ralph Baric and Shi Zhengli-Li at the University of North Carolina and the Wuhan Institute of Virology, respectively.

Above and beyond the money trail leading to Peter Daszak, Dr. Fauci's NIAID has awarded 173 grants to Dr. Ralph S. Baric for his research. According to Dr. Fauci, Dr. Baric—despite what you read earlier in the book—is not doing Gain-of-Function research:

> Dr. Baric is not doing gain-of-function research, and if it is, it is according to the guidelines and is being conducted in North Carolina. If you look at the grant and if you look at the progress reports, it is not gain-of-function, despite the fact that people tweet that, write about it.[106]

Given the published papers and patents, it is clear that Dr. Fauci, the NIAID, and other federal agencies and their heads have funded Gain-of-Function research, which has not only been published but has resulted in patents being issued. Patents that produce financial benefits for these agencies and include potential personal, professional, and financial benefits for their department heads. In addition to the materials we have already considered, there are clearly potential conflicts of interest (COI) with the vaccines currently under EUA by the FDA. For example, NIAID Ref. No. 2015-33448, page 105, shows one such potential conflict of interest, where NIAID and Moderna jointly own and developed an mRNA vaccine. The NIAID document shows the Moderna drug vaccine research was being transferred to the University of North Carolina at Chapel Hill, where Dr. Ralph S. Baric is professor.[107]

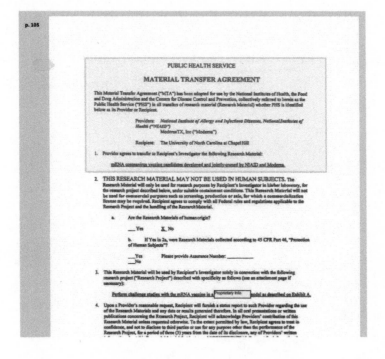

Collectively these documents reveal, as shown in the appendix, that more than $61 million dollars in research funding was paid to Peter Daszak at EcoHealth, who then worked with Ralph S. Baric at the University of North Carolina, and Shi Zhengli at the Wuhan Institute of Virology, to conduct research on viruses including Gain-of-Function research on coronaviruses.

CHAPTER 4

The SARS-CoV-2 Gain-of-Function Smoking Gun Is the Spike Protein

Coronaviruses are so named for the corona (Latin for crown) that surrounds the outer surface of the virus. A transmission electron microscope image of SARS-CoV-2 shows the virus with the crown of spike proteins emanating from its membrane.[1] The following electron micrograph of coronaviruses both attaching to and inside human lung cells shows the typical spike protein crown appearance that gives the virus the family name coronaviridae or coronavirus.[2]

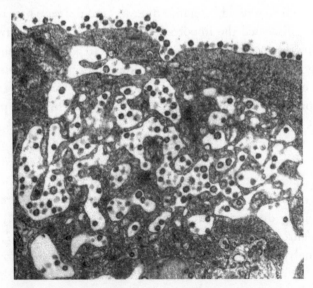

Refer again to the first image of the color photo insert. Enlargement of the spike protein, showing its molecular structure and critical components following Gain-of-Function changes discussed in previous chapters, is shown in that figure.

In 2015, Dr. Fang Li wrote a mini review—funded by NIH grant RO1AI089728—discussing the importance of recognizing not only the C-terminal domain of the S1 part of the spike protein but also the N-terminal domain (NTD).[3] Included in this review was the importance of DPP4 and its role in inflammation and the release of cytokines, as well as the importance of Transmissible Gastroenteritis Virus (TGEV) that Baric mutated to make the virus infectious in 2000 as discussed earlier in this book. The NTD of TGEV is particularly problematic because this region of the spike protein recognizes N-glycolylneuraminic acid (Neu5Gc), which we have previously raised as a concern, explaining the "inflammation" associated with certain animal products.[4] Others have echoed that concern.[5]

Before addressing the specific inserts and resulting conformational change of the spike protein, it is important to understand that the formation of antibodies is not always a good thing. The process as I originally explained in the "Inflammation and Heart Disease Theory" can also be harmful—particularly from the right type of an invading virus. However, sometimes those antibodies, in the case of *Streptococcus pneumoniae* (strep throat), can cause damage to the valves of your heart, producing rheumatic heart disease. In other instances, as in the formation of antibodies to the N-terminal of SARS-CoV-2, it can enhance the infectivity of the virus by a factor of four to tenfold,[6] enhance disease,[7] and decrease patient survival.[8]

Having discussed the importance of TMPRSS2 previously and those involved in discovering this, it is important to know that this enzyme, which is genetically coded for, plays an important role in the susceptibility of people exposed to SARS-CoV-2. Once the receptor-binding domain of the spike protein attaches to the ACE2 receptor, the TMPRSS2 protease cell receptor is brought into play. Both ACE2 and TMPRSS2 are key determinants for entry of the virus.[9]

Since all proteins and structures in our body are coded for based upon our specific genetic makeup, the specificity of SARS-CoV-2 and the series of receptors it uses to sequentially enter our cells are critical to understanding differences in susceptibility. We have already discussed the genes/chromosomes involved with ACE2 and TMPRSS2. However, further analysis into ACE2 and TMPRSS2 shows considerable differences between races:

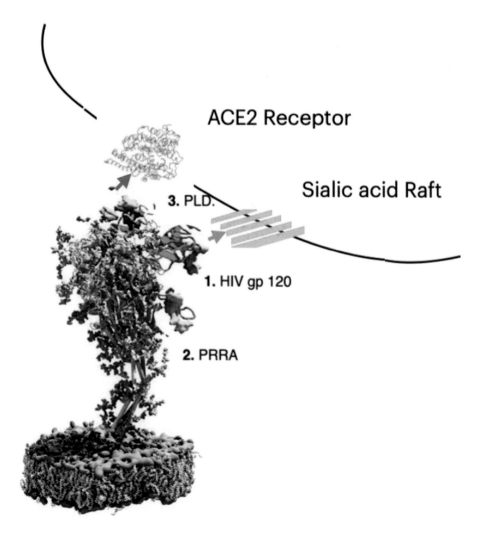

ACE2 Receptor

Sialic acid Raft

3. PLD.

1. HIV gp 120

2. PRRA

```
                                          S1/S2                              S2'
Human SARS-CoV BJ01              655 - GICASYHTVSLL----RSTS - 670    790 - DPLKPTKRSFIED - 802
Human SARS-CoV CUHK-W1           655 - GICASYHTVSLL----RSTS - 670    790 - DPLKPTKRSFIED - 802
Human SARS-CoV Tor2              655 - GICASYHTVSLL----RSTS - 670    790 - DPLKPTKRSFIED - 802
Human SARS-CoV Frankfurt-1       655 - GICASYHTVSLL----RSTS - 670    790 - DPLKPTKRSFIED - 802
Human SARS-CoV Urbani            655 - GICASYHTVSLL----RSTS - 670    790 - DPLKPTKRSFIED - 802
Civet SARS-CoV civet020          655 - GICASYHTVSSL----RSTS - 670    790 - DPLKPTKRSFIED - 802
Civet SARS-CoV SZ16              655 - GICASYHTVSSL----RSTS - 670    790 - DPLKPTKRSFIED - 802
Raccoon dog SARS-CoV A030        655 - GICASYHTVSSL----RSTS - 670    790 - DPLKPTKRSFIED - 802
SARS-CoV-2                      (669 - GICASYQTQTNSPRRARSVA - 688)   808 - DPSKPSKRSFIED - 820
Pangolin CoV MP789               n/a - GICASYQTQTNS----RSVS - n/a    n/a - DPSKPSKRSFIED - n/a
Bat SARSr-CoV RaTG13             669 - GICASYQTQTNS----RSVA - 684    804 - DPSKPSKRSFIED - 816
Bat SARSr-CoV LYRa11             659 - GICASYHTASLL----RNTD - 674    794 - DPLKPTKRSFIED - 806
Bat SARSr-CoV LYRa3              659 - GICASYHTASLL----RNTG - 674    794 - DPLKPTKRSFIED - 806
Bat SARSr-CoV RsSHC014           656 - GICASYHTVSSL----RSTS - 671    791 - DPLKPTKRSFIED - 803
Bat SARSr-CoV Rs4084             656 - GICASYHTVSSL----RSTS - 671    791 - DPLKPTKRSFIED - 803
Bat SARSr-CoV WIV1               656 - GICASYHTVSSL----RSTS - 671    791 - DPLKPTKRSFIED - 803
Bat SARSr-CoV Rs3367             656 - GICASYHTVSSL----RSTS - 671    791 - DPLKPTKRSFIED - 803
Bat SARSr-CoV Rs7327             656 - GICASYHTVSSL----RSTS - 671    791 - DPLKPTKRSFIED - 803
Bat SARSr-CoV Rs9401             656 - GICASYHTVSSL----RSTS - 671    791 - DPLKPTKRSFIED - 803
Bat SARSr-CoV Rs4231             655 - GICASYHTVSSL----RSTS - 670    790 - DPLKPTKRSFIED - 802
Bat SARSr-CoV WIV16              655 - GICASYHTVSSL----RSTS - 670    790 - DPLKPTKRSFIED - 802
Bat SARSr-CoV Rs4874             655 - GICASYHTVSSL----RSTS - 670    790 - DPLKPTKRSFIED - 802
Bat SARSr-CoV ZC45               646 - GICASYHTASIL----RSTS - 661    781 - DPSKPSKRSFIED - 793
Bat SARSr-CoV ZXC21              645 - GICASYHTASIL----RSTG - 660    780 - DPSKPSKRSFIED - 792
Bat SARSr-CoV Rf4092             634 - GICASYHTASTL----RGVG - 649    769 - DPSKPTKRSFIED - 781
Bat SARSr-CoV Rf/JL2012          636 - GICASYHTASLL----RSTG - 651    771 - DPLKPTKRSFIED - 783
Bat SARSr-CoV JTMC15             636 - GICASYHTASLL----RSTG - 651    771 - DPLKPTKRSFIED - 783
Bat SARSr-CoV 16B0133            636 - GICASYHTASLL----RSTG - 651    771 - DPLKPTKRSFIED - 783
Bat SARSr-CoV B15-21             636 - GICASYHTASLL----RSTG - 651    771 - DPLKPTKRSFIED - 783
Bat SARSr-CoV YN2013             633 - GICASYHTASTL----RSIG - 648    768 - DPSKPTKRSFIED - 780
Bat SARSr-CoV Anlong-103         633 - GICASYHTASTL----RSVG - 648    768 - DPSKPTKRSFIED - 780
Bat SARSr-CoV Rp/Shaanxi2011     640 - GICASYHTASVL----RSTG - 655    775 - DPSKPTKRSFIED - 787
Bat SARSr-CoV Rs/HuB2013         641 - GICASYHTASVL----RSTG - 656    776 - DPSKPTKRSFIED - 788
Bat SARSr-CoV YNLF/34C           641 - GICASYHTASVL----RSTG - 656    776 - DPLKPTKRSFIED - 788
Bat SARSr-CoV YNLF/31C           641 - GICASYHTASVL----RSTG - 656    776 - DPLKPTKRSFIED - 788
Bat SARSr-CoV Rf1                641 - GICASYHTASHL----RSTG - 656    776 - DPLKPTKRSFIED - 788
Bat SARSr-CoV 273                641 - GICASYHTASLL----RSTG - 656    776 - DPLKPTKRSFIED - 788
Bat SARSr-CoV Rf/SX2013          639 - GICASYHTASLL----RSTG - 654    774 - DPLKPTKRSFIED - 786
Bat SARSr-CoV Rf/HeB2013         641 - GICASYHTASLL----RSTG - 656    776 - DPLKPTKRSFIED - 788
Bat SARSr-CoV Cp/Yunnan2011      641 - GICASYHTASTL----RNTG - 656    776 - DPSKPTKRSFIED - 788
Bat SARSr-CoV Rs672              641 - GICASYHTASTL----RSVG - 656    776 - DPSKPTKRSFIED - 788
Bat SARSr-CoV Rs4255             641 - GICASYHTASTL----RSVG - 656    776 - DPSKPTKRSFIED - 788
Bat SARSr-CoV Rs4081             641 - GICASYHTASTL----RSVG - 656    776 - DPSKPTKRSFIED - 788
Bat SARSr-CoV Rm1                641 - GICASYHTASVL----RSTG - 656    776 - DPSKPTKRSFIED - 788
Bat SARSr-CoV 279                641 - GICASYHTASVL----RSTG - 656    776 - DPSKPTKRSFIED - 788
Bat SARSr-CoV Rs/GX2013          642 - GICASYHTASLL----RSTG - 657    777 - DPSKPTKRSFIED - 789
Bat SARSr-CoV Rs806              641 - GICASYHTASLL----RSTG - 656    777 - DPSKPTKRSFIED - 788
Bat SARSr-CoV HKU3-1             642 - GICASYHTASVL----RSTG - 657    777 - DPSKPTKRSFIED - 789
Bat SARSr-CoV Longquan-140       642 - GICASYHTASTL----RSTG - 657    777 - DPSKPTKRSFIED - 789
Bat SARSr-CoV Rp3                641 - GICASYHTASTL----RSVG - 656    776 - DPSKPTKRSFIED - 788
Bat SARSr-CoV Rs4247             642 - GICASYHTASTL----RSVG - 657    777 - DPSKPTKRSFIED - 789
Bat SARSr-CoV Rs4237             641 - GICASYHTASTL----RSVG - 656    776 - DPSKPTKRSFIED - 788
Bat SARSr-CoV As6526             641 - GICASYHTASTL----RSVG - 656    777 - DPSKPTKRSFIED - 789
Bat SARSr-CoV BtKY72/KEN         660 - GICAKFGS---D----KIRMG - 673    793 - DPKKLSYRSFIED - 805
Bat SARSr-CoV BM48-31            658 - GICAKYTNVSST---LVRSG - 674    794 - DPAKPSSRSFIED - 806
                                       ****.:                             ** * ; ******


Alpha    HCoV-NL63               735 - GICADGSLI----FVRPFNSS - 751    860 - FNIRSSRIAGRSAIED - 875
Alpha    HCoV-229E               554 - GVCADGSII----AVQPFNVS - 570    679 - LPTSGSNVAGRSAIED - 694
Beta 2a  HCoV-OC43               753 - GYCVDYSK-----NRPSIGAI - 768    901 - LGSECSKASSRSAIED - 916
Beta 2a  HCoV-HKU1               742 - GFCVDYNSPSSSSRRRRFSI - 762    895 - LGPRCGS-SSRSFFED - 909
Beta 2b  SARS-CoV                655 - GICASYHTVS-L----LRSTS - 670    790 - DP---LKPTKRSFIED - 802
Beta 2b  SARS-CoV-2              669 - GICASYQTQT-NSPRRARSVA - 688    808 - DP---SRPSKRSFIED - 820
Beta 2c  MERS-CoV                734 - SLCALPDTPSTLTPRSVRSVP - 754    877 - VSISTGSRSARSAIED - 892
                                       . *              *                 ; ** :**
```

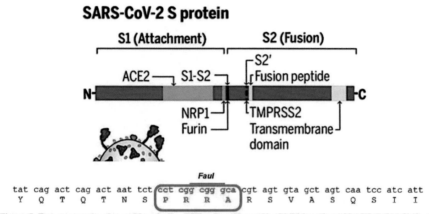

Figure 7. Two consecutive Arg residues in the -PRRA- insertion at the S1/S2 junction of SARS-CoV-2 Spike are both coded by a rare codon, CGG. *A FauI restriction site, 5'-(N)₆GCGGG-3', is embedded in the coding sequence of the "inserted" PRRA segment, which may be used as a marker to monitor the preservation of the introduced furin-cleavage site.*

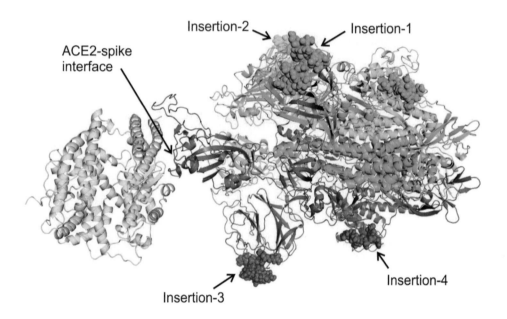

COVID_19 "Exogeneous Informative Elements"

HIV2C
HIV-1 isolate 07.RU.SP.R497.VI.G3 from Russia
envelope glycoprotein (env) gene
32/39 82%

```
TTGTTATTAAAGTAT TT --- TTTCAATTTTGTACTTATC
III IIIIIII IIII I I I   II IIII IIIIII II I III
TTGTTATTAAAGTCTGTGAATTTCAATTTTGTAATGATC
```

HIV2B
Human immunodeficiency virus type 2 complete genome from strain HIV-2UC1
22/26 85%

```
TGTTTATTTTGCTCCTAGTTATTAAGT
IIIIIIIIIIIIII I III I IIII
TGTTTATTTTGCTTCCACTTAGAAGT
```

HIV1A
HIV-1 isolate 19663.24H9 fro...
Netherlands envelope glycoprotein env
gene
25/28 89%

```
AATGGTACTAAGAGGGTAGATAAC ACTG
II IIIIIIIIII II II I   II IIII  III
AATGGTACTAAGAGGTT TGATAAC CCTG
```

HIV1B
HIV-1 isolate 4045_Plasma_Visir1 _amplicon5a from Malawi envelope glycoprotein (env) gene
28/32 88%

```
CGGTACTAAT--GTTACTAACCCTAGTAATGTT
IIIIIIII II IIII IIII IIIIIIIIIII
CGGTACTTATTGTTAAATAACGCTACTAAGGTT
```

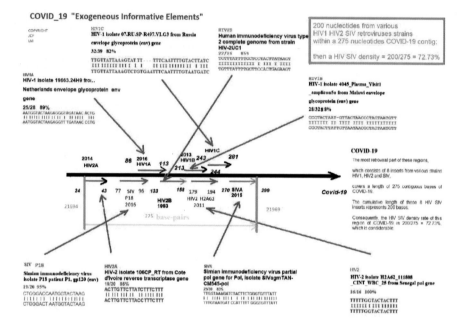

COVID-19

The most retroviral part of these regions,

which consists of 8 inserts from various strains HIV1, HIV2 and SIV,

covers a length of 275 contiguous bases of COVID-19.

The cumulative length of these 8 HIV SIV inserts represents 200 bases.

Consequently, the HIV SIV density rate of this region of COVID-19 is 200/275 = 72.73%, which is considerable.

200 nucleotides from various HIV1 HIV2 SIV retroviruses strains within a 275 nucleotides COVID-19 contig;

then a HIV SIV density = 200/275 = 72.73%

SIV P18
Simian immunodeficiency virus isolate P18 patient P1, gp120 (env)
19/20 95%

```
CTGGGACCAATGGTACTAAG
IIIIII I IIIIIIIIIII
CTGGGACT AATGGTACTAAG
```

HIV2A
HIV-2 isolate 106CP_RT from Cote d'Ivoire reverse transcriptase gene
19/20 95%

```
ACTTGTTCTTATCTTTCTTT
II IIII III II  II IIII III
ACTTGTTCTTACCTTTCTTT
```

SIVA
Simian immunodeficiency virus partial pol gene for Pol, isolate SIVagmTAN-CM545-pol
25/30 83%

```
TTGGTAAAGATCTACTTCTGGGTGTTTATT
II IIII IIII I  II IIIIIIIIIIII
TTTGTAATGAT CCATTTT GGGTGTTTATT
```

HIV2
HIV-2 isolate H2A62_111808 _CINT_WBC_25 from Senegal pol gene
16/16 100%

```
TTTTTGGTACTACTTT
IIIIIII I III IIIIII
TTTTTGGTACTACTTT
```

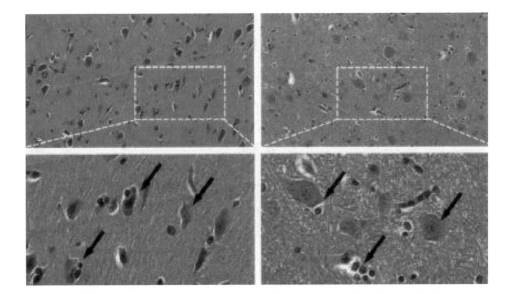

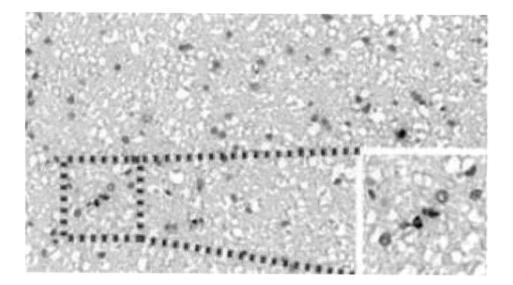

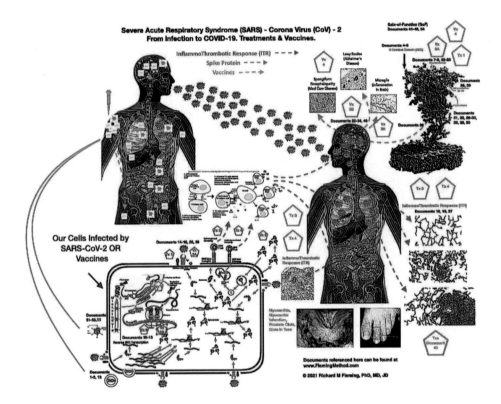

Severe Acute Respiratory Syndrome (SARS) - Corona Virus (CoV) - 2
From Infection to COVID-19. Treatments & Vaccines.

Documents referenced here can be found at
www.FlemingMethod.com

© 2021 Richard M Fleming, PhD, MD, JD

> We found that **ACE2 polymorphisms** were more likely to be associated with cardiovascular and pulmonary conditions by altering the angiotensinogen-ACE2 interactions, such as p.Arg514- Gly in the African/African-American population. Unique but prevalent polymorphisms in **TMPRSS2**, including p.Val160Met (rs12329760), may provide potential explanations for differential genetic susceptibility to COVID-19 as well as for risk factors, including cancer and the high-risk group of male patients.[10] [Emphasis added.]

In fact, the expression of TMPRSS2 is significantly greater in black individuals than any other race, as shown in the following graphic.[11]

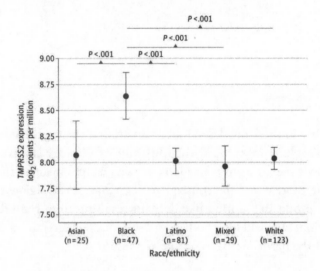

While we know there has been considerable effort by Peter Daszak to downplay the Gain-of-Function origin of SARS-CoV-2—given that he would undoubtedly lose his funding from the US government if concerns were raised—his communications[12] with individuals, including Dr. Linfa Wang from Duke-National University of Singapore (NUS) Medical School and Dr. Ralph Baric of the University of North Carolina, show Daszak's efforts to distance himself from Wang and Baric, who have collaborated with Dr. Shi Zhengli of the Wuhan Institute of Virology for many years. The following was obtained with a FOIA request by U.S. Right to Know.[13]

As shown in the last two chapters, the United States federal government paid for Gain-of-Function and gene manipulation research and is included in the patents of this work. Its role in the development of SARS-CoV-2 demonstrates its culpability—both criminally and civilly—for the harm

To: Peter Daszak[daszak@ecohealthalliance.org]; Baric, Toni C[antoinette_baric@med.unc.edu]
Cc: Alison Andre[andre@ecohealthalliance.org]; Aleksei Chmura[chmura@ecohealthalliance.org]
From: Baric, Ralph S[/O=EXCHANGELABS/OU=EXCHANGE ADMINISTRATIVE GROUP
(FYDIBOHF23SPDLT)/CN=RECIPIENTS/CN=BB0D9CC80C184735A4E862C3BDD8A15D-RALPH S BAR]
Sent: Thur 2/6/2020 4:01:22 PM (UTC-05:00)
Subject: RE: No need for you to sign the "Statement" Ralph!!

I also think this is a good decision. Otherwise it looks self-serving and we lose impact. ralph

---

From: Peter Daszak <daszak@ecohealthalliance.org>
Sent: Thursday, February 6, 2020 3:16 PM
To: Baric, Ralph S <rbaric@email.unc.edu>; Baric, Toni C <antoinette_baric@med.unc.edu>
Cc: Alison Andre <andre@ecohealthalliance.org>; Aleksei Chmura <chmura@ecohealthalliance.org>
Subject: No need for you to sign the "Statement" Ralph!!
Importance: High

I spoke with Linfa last night about the statement we sent round. He thinks, and I agree with him, that you, me and him should not
sign this statement, so it has some distance from us and therefore doesn't work in a counterproductive way.

Jim Hughes, Linda Saif, Hume Field, and I believe Rita Colwell will sign it, then I'll send it round some other key people tonight.
We'll then put it out in a way that doesn't link it back to our collaboration so we maximize an independent voice.

Cheers,

Peter

Peter Daszak
President

EcoHealth Alliance
460 West 34th Street – 17th Floor
New York, NY 10001

done not only in the United States but also around the world, independent of the virus's release from the Wuhan Institute of Virology laboratory.

It is now time for us to take a look at two changes made to the SARS-CoV-2 spike protein and the consequential change at the regional binding site (RBS), producing a prion-like domain resulting from the PRRA and HIV insertions. We will look both at the evidence of this Gain-of-Function change and the harm caused to people as a result.

PROLINE-ARGININE-ARGININE-ALANINE (PRRA) INSERT

Following the attachment of the SARS-CoV-2 spike protein to the ACE2 receptor and then the TMPRSS2 site, the spike protein undergoes a special type of protein cleavage. This step is essential for SARS-CoV-2 to infect humans,[14] and it is related to the spread of the virus from cell to cell and the virulence of the virus.

This furin (PRRA) cleavage site has been shown to be critical for other viruses, including avian influenza virus and Newcastle disease virus, and it has *not* been found in any other influenza or coronavirus.[15]

As shown in the color figure images, the PRRA insert is *not* present in any other coronavirus on the planet.[16] The furin cleavage site lies in the stable part of the spike protein—the S1 component. Most if not all of the mutations being seen in SARS-CoV-2 are occurring in the S2 component of the Spike Protein.

A final point of interest lies in ownership and patent rights for inserting furin protease cleavage sites in membranes.[17] The patent specifically states, "This protocol can be used to produce virus membrane protein domains for structural analysis and for trials as vaccines."

We also know that the PRRA furin cleavage site is involved in the conversion of the HIV envelope precursor glycoprotein (gp) 160 cleavage[18] to gp120 for HIV virus assembly.[19] That leads us to our next Gain-of-Function: HIV gp120.

INSERTION OF FURIN PROTEASE CLEAVAGE SITES IN MEMBRANE PROTEINS AND USES THEREOF

CROSS-REFERENCE TO RELATED APPLICATION

This non-provisional patent application claims benefit of provisional patent application U.S. Ser. No. 60/469,126, filed May 9, 2003, now abandoned.

The United States government may own certain rights to this invention pursuant to grant number AI 42775 from the National Institutes of Health.

HIV GLYCOPROTEIN 120 (HIV GP 120)

The second Gain-of-Function insert[20] we have evidence of includes the HIV-gp 120. As shown in the first figure of the color insert, the gp120 insert in the spike protein, is larger than the PRRA insert.

We know that Shi Zhengli-Li admitted to working with the spike protein of coronaviruses following the initial outbreak in 2002 with the specific intent of increasing the ability of SARS-CoV to infect people.[21]

We now know that HIV gp120 attaches to the sialic acid receptor raft and is associated with the inflammation and blood clotting first described by myself in 1994, as discussed previously in this book, and that the gp120 is not only involved in this InflammoThrombotic Response (COVID-19) but also prion diseases.[22]

We also know that in 2002 when Zhengli was manipulating the Spike Protein and working with the HIV gp120 pseudovirus with her SARS-CoV-1 coronavirus Gain-of-Function research, that it was known that HIV gp120 itself was understood to cause prion brain diseases.[23]

In 2010, Zhengli and colleagues began investigating ACE2 receptors.[24] It had previously been shown that:

> the angiotensin converting enzyme 2 (ACE2) protein, a known SARS-CoV receptor, from a horseshoe bat was unable to act as a functional receptor for SARS-CoV.[25]

Using the HIV-based pseudovirus and live SARS-CoV-1 infection assays, Zhengli and others were able to prove that if "several key residues" of the spike protein were "altered," they could increase infectivity.

In 2013, Zhengli-Li[26] began working with Ralph Baric[27] on the HKU4 spike protein of the MERS coronavirus, the very type of research that led to the shutdown of Gain-of-Function research in 2014:[28]

> Reengineered HKU4 spike, aiming to build its capacity to mediate viral entry into human cells. To this end, we introduced two single mutations. . . . Mutations in these motifs in coronavirus spikes have demonstrated dramatic effects on viral entry into human cells. (Funded by NIH Grants RO1AI089728 and RO1AI110700.)

The subsequent presentation made by Zhengli at the Shanghai Jiao Tong University on November 14, 2018, titled "Studies on Bat Coronavirus and Its Cross-Species Infection" has since been deleted from the university's website.

Following Zhengli's 2002 work and prior to her work with the HKU4 spike protein, Zhengli and others at the Wuhan Institute of Virology used the HIV-based pseudovirus to prove that SARS-like coronavirus (SL-CoV) was *unable* to infect human cells or the cells of horseshoe bats:

> In this study, a human immunodeficiency virus (HIV)-based pseudovirus system was employed to address these issues. Our results indicated that the SL-CoV S protein is unable to use ACE2 proteins of different species for cell entry and that SARS-CoV S protein also failed to bind the ACE2 molecule of the horseshoe bat, Rhinolophus pearsonii.[29]

They went on to state the inability of these viruses to infect cells using the ACE2 receptor regardless of its origin.

> Our results indicated that the bat SL-CoV (Rp3) S protein is unable to use ACE2 for cell entry regardless of the origin of the ACE2 molecule. We also demonstrated that the human SARS-CoV S cannot use bat RpACE2 as a functional receptor.

Genetic manipulation (Gain-of-Function) made it possible for the hybrid S (spike) protein to infect cells:

> However, when the RBD of SL-CoV S was replaced with that from the SARS-CoV S, the hybrid S protein was able to use the huACE2 for cell entry.

In 2009, Chinese researchers showed that the SARS-CoV-1 spike protein included fusion glycoproteins[30] found in class I viral glycoproteins[31] such as found in HIV.[32] According to Dr. Li Meng Yan, SARS-CoV-1 was also a bioweapon developed by the Chinese Communist Party (CCP).[33]

As discussed previously, we know that furin (PRRA) cleavage is responsible not only for increasing the infectivity of SARS-CoV-2 but also for converting HIV gp160 to gp120 and gp41, demonstrating its role in HIV infections and any potential inserts of HIV material (as discussed previously). This raises additional concerns about the combination of PRRA and HIV gp120 inserts.

We also know from the work of Pradhan and others—currently under revision—that his research team found what they considered to be four unique inserts into the SARS-CoV-2 spike protein.[34]

Dr. Zhang et al. analyzed these four inserts comparing these genetic sequences to known sequences of other viruses using Basic Local Alignment Search Tool (BLAST).[35] The color photo insert shows the ACE2 receptor in yellow, with insertions 1 through 4 identified as shown.

The investigators concluded that three of the four inserts are present in other coronaviruses:

> Among the 4 "insertions" (ISs) of the 2019-nCoV, IS1 has only 1 residue different from the bat coronavirus, and 3 out of 7 residues are identical with MERS-CoV. IS2 and IS3 are all identical to the bat coronavirus. For **IS4**, although the local sequence alignment by BLAST **did not hit the bat coronavirus** in Table 4, it has a close evolutionary relation with the bat coronavirus in the MSA. In particular, the first 6 residues in the IS4 fragment "QTQTNS**PRRA**" from 2019-nCoV are identical to the bat CoV, while **the last 4 residues, which were absent in the bat coronavirus or SARS-CoV,**

have at least 50% identity to MERS-CoV and HCoV-HKU1.[36] [Emphasis added.]

Taken together, these statements from research paid for by NIAID (AI134678) and the National Science Foundation (DBI1564756, IIS1901191)—both agencies involved in the funding of Daszak, Baric, and Zhengli Gain-of-Function research—appear to confirm both Dr. Li-Meng Yan's assertion[37] that SARS-CoV-1 was the first bioweapon and that SARS-CoV-2 is the advanced version noting the **PRRA** segment.

Finally, we turn our attention to Professor Luc Montagnier—the discoverer of Human Immunodeficiency Virus (HIV).[38] Montagnier has published one paper[39] and has submitted another for consideration.[40] In both of these papers, Montagnier utilizes the same BLAST technology for analysis of the genetic code of SARS-CoV-2.

He notes eighteen RNA fragments similar to HIV or simian (higher primates) that have the potential to change the genetic expression of COVID-19:

> 18 RNA fragments of homology equal or more than 80% with human or simian retroviruses have been found in the COVID_19 genome. These fragments are 18 to 30 nucleotides long and therefore have the potential to modify the gene expression of Covid19. We have named them external Informative Elements or EIE. These EIE are not dispersed randomly, but are concentrated in a small part of the genome.[41]

This is shown schematically in the color figure labelled Exogenous Informative Elements.[42]

As stated so eloquently by Montagnier, the spike protein not only has the PRRA insertion (twelve nucleotide bases) but also a 1770 nucleotide[43] base (590 amino acid) insertion matching HIV-1:

> We have studied the most recent genetic evolution of the COVID_19 strains involved in the world epidemic. We found a significant occurrence of mutations and deletions in the 225 bases area.
>
> On sampling genomes, we show that this 225 bases key region of each genome, rich in EIE, and the 1770 bases SPIKE region evolve much faster than the corresponding whole genome (cases of 44 patients' genomes from WA Seattle state, original epicenter in USA).

In the comparative analysis of both SPIKES genes of COVID_19 and Bat RaTG13 we note two abnormal facts:

1) the insertion of 4 contiguous PRRA amino acids in the middle of SPIKE (we show that this site was already an optimal cleavage site BEFORE this insertion).

2) an abnormal distribution of synonymous codons in the second half of SPIKE.

Finally we show the insertion in this 1770 bases SPIKE region of a significant pair of EIEs from Plasmodium Yoelii and of a possible HIV1 EIE with a crucial SPIKE mutation.[44]

As pointed out by Yan, this type of Gain-of-Function gene editing has made it possible to create novel coronaviruses possessing unique properties![45]

PRION-LIKE DOMAIN (PLD) AT THE REGIONAL BINDING SITE (RBS)

When a structure has pressure exerted upon it, that structure will change its shape. For example, if you have a box and you press in on the corner of the box, you will change the shape of the box. With the insertion of nucleotides (pushing on the box) into the spike protein (the box), the shape of the spike protein (box) will change. The insertion of PRRA and HIV gp120 subsequently causes a conformation shape of the molecule known as the SARS-CoV-2 spike protein. This conformational change has resulted in the development of, in addition to any HIV insertions (e.g. gp120), an area with prion-like properties, that is, a prion-like domain (PLD), where the spike protein attaches to the ACE2 receptor. This area is known as the regional binding site (RBS) as shown in the color figure of the Spike protein.

The Vaccine Adverse Events Reporting System (VAERS) cosponsored by the CDC, the Food and Drug Administration (FDA), and the HHS has been inundated with adverse events following the widespread vaccination of American citizens under the Emergency Use Authorization (EUA) implementation of the Pfizer, Moderna, and Johnson & Johnson (Janssen) experimental drug vaccines. The implementation of these EUA drugs are the direct result of the secretary of HHS and FDA actions.[46]

The Harvard vaccine injury study[47] submitted to the Agency for Healthcare Research and Quality (AHRQ) reported that less than 0.3 percent of all adverse drug events are reported, with 1 percent to 13 percent percent of all serious events reported. The study concluded that less than 1 percent of all vaccine adverse events are reported.

Despite these limitations in reporting, when the Swine Flu vaccine[48] of the mid-1970s produced neurologic damage, including Guillain-Barré syndrome,[49] following the first twenty-five deaths, the swine flu vaccine and vaccination program were stopped by the US government.

Today the VAERS reporting system—despite the absence of an ICD-10 code for physicians to report adverse events to the SARS-CoV-2 drug vaccines, inability of physicians to leave verbal or electronic reports of adverse events, and electronic reports being "kicked out" of the system, VAERS still shows thousands of deaths following SARS-CoV-2 vaccination, with many more experiencing neurologic and InflammoThrombotic Response (ITR) including heart damage, spontaneous abortions, and other harm resulting from the vaccinations.[50] By contrast, twenty-five deaths stopped the swine flu vaccine of the mid-1970s.

While the explanation for these ITRs has been extensively explained[51] and confirmed in patients dying from COVID-19,[52] the reason for the neurologic damage can be seen in the animal studies looking at the consequences of the SARS-CoV-2 spike protein resulting either from person-to-person spread of the virus or from the drug vaccines, which easily crosses the blood-brain barrier (BBB),[53] as do the lipid nanoparticles[54] used in the Pfizer and Moderna vaccines.

These spike proteins—independent of whether they are the result of person-to-person transfer or vaccination resulting in billions of mRNA or dsDNA coding for the spike protein—have prion-like domains (PLD) in the region of the Regional Binding Domain (RBD) as well as any HIV gp120 insertion. As already noted, the RBD is that part of the spike protein that attaches to the ACE2 receptor on human cells to begin the infection and potential ITR and prion disease (e.g. spongeform encephalopathy/mad cow disease; Lewy body/Alzheimer disease, etc.), with short- and long-term sequelae. Evidence is mounting that these prion diseases are causing heart and brain damage.

Two published papers looking at the consequences of the SARS-CoV-2 spike protein penetrating the brain of humanized mice[55] and rhesus macaques[56] show brain inflammation, mad cow disease, and Alzheimer disease.

In the humanized mice (mice that are genetically altered to provide a human ACE2 receptor to allow the researchers to look at what the virus does once it infects cells), following infection with the spike protein, 95 percent of the animals died after two weeks. The remaining two animals were then euthanized, and the brains of the animals were examined:

> Despite infection and moderate **inflammation** in the **lungs, lethality was invariably associated with viral neuroinvasion and neuronal damage** (including spinal motor neurons). Neuroinvasion occurred following virus transport through the **olfactory** neuroepithelium. [Emphasis added.]

In other words, even though all of the mice showed damaging inflammation in their lungs, all the animals died due to brain damage with the virus entering the brain through the olfactory (sense of smell) system.

The images[57] included in the color photo section show the brains of rhesus macaque monkeys infected with SARS-CoV-2 after the virus was introduced through the olfactory system (nose).

As shown in the microscopic slide in the color insert, once infected the brain cells take on the appearance of a sponge. When this happens, the resulting disease is called *Spongiform encephalopathy* (sponge-like brain), a.k.a. mad cow disease.

A second group of research scientists in the Netherlands also looked at the brains of Rhesus macaques[58] following infection with SARS-CoV-2 spike proteins. This group of research scientists found inflammation and Lewy body changes using Positron Emission Tomography (PET) nuclear imaging applying semi-quantitative[59] methods. The brains of these animals demonstrated increased metabolic activity in the brain five to six weeks after brain infection.

Microscopic examination of the brains of these animals showed "infection" and "overactivation of the immune system" revealing both microglia and CD3 inflammatory cells. These brains also showed Lewy bodies seen in Alzheimer disease, Parkinson's disease, and a variety of other neuromuscular diseases.[60]

Recognition of these neurologic problems along with concerns about the origins[61] of SARS-CoV-2 have been raised by many individuals, not the least of whom is neurobiologist Kevin W. McCairn, PhD, who currently lives in Japan. Dr. McCairn is one of the world's preeminent experts in primate behavior and neurologic diseases.

It is critical to understand that it makes no difference whether the spike protein[62] is introduced into the body via person-to-person transfer or via injection[63] of biologicals as shown in the color insert.[64] The only difference appears to be in the number of mRNA or dsDNA molecules introduced into someone (antigenic load), which can either be found by reading through the EUA documents[65] or calculated using well-established methods. For the mRNA vaccines, this results in 13.1 billion[66] mRNAs and, for the dsDNA, 50 billion.

CHAPTER 5

An Intentionally Released Bioweapon

All too often, people believe that weapons are designed to kill people. I would argue quite the contrary. The best weapon doesn't kill people; it devastates and demoralizes them. It reduces their will and capacity to wage war or to fight back. In battle, the best way to do that is to maim the enemy so their friends will come to their aid and leave the battlefield to shelter their friend.

The best weapon to devastate a country is one that removes the will of the people to fight. It effectively diminishes the lifestyles of the enemy, reducing the security of life as the enemy knows it and replaces that security and freedom with fear and uncertainty. SARS-CoV-2 has done exactly that. It has devastated economies, removed the personal freedoms people were used to, reduced goods and services, and turned friends against friends and family members against family members. It has divided nations and people.

According to the Biological Weapons Convention (BWC) treaty, it is a violation of the treaty—signed and ratified by the United States—to develop, acquire, retain, or produce any biological agent that has no justification for prevention or peaceful purposes, and any use of such biological weapons or toxins is to be "condemned."[1]

The Biological Weapons Convention (BWC) At A Glance

FACT SHEETS & BRIEFS

Last Reviewed: March 2020

Contact: Daryl Kimball, *Executive Director,* (202) 463-8270 x107

The Biological Weapons Convention (BWC) is a legally binding treaty that outlaws biological arms. After being discussed and negotiated in the United Nations' disarmament forum starting in 1969, the BWC opened for signature on April 10, 1972, and entered into force on March 26, 1975. It currently has 183 states-parties, including Palestine, and four signatories (Egypt, Haiti, Somalia, Syria, and Tanzania). Ten states have neither signed nor ratified the BWC (Chad, Comoros, Djibouti, Eritrea, Israel, Kiribati, Micronesia, Namibia, South Sudan and Tuvalu).

Terms of the Treaty

The BWC bans:

- The development, stockpiling, acquisition, retention, and production of:
  1. Biological agents and toxins "of types and in quantities that have no justification for prophylactic, protective or other peaceful purposes;"
  2. Weapons, equipment, and delivery vehicles "designed to use such agents or toxins for hostile purposes or in armed conflict."
- The transfer of or assistance with acquiring the agents, toxins, weapons, equipment, and delivery vehicles described above.

The convention further requires states-parties to destroy or divert to peaceful purposes the "agents, toxins, weapons, equipment, and means of delivery" described above within nine months of the convention's entry into force. The BWC does not ban the use of biological and toxin weapons but reaffirms the 1925 Geneva Protocol, which prohibits such use. It also does not ban biodefense programs.

Seventh Review Conference

The seventh BWC review conference was held in December 2011. The Final Declaration document concluded that "under all circumstances the use of bacteriological (biological) and toxin weapons is effectively prohibited by the Convention and affirms the determination of States parties to condemn any use of biological agents or toxins other than for peaceful purposes, by anyone at any time."

United States Federal Code 12 U.S.C. Chapter 10 § 175 expressly prohibits such biological weapons and makes it a criminal offense:[2]

§175. Prohibitions with respect to biological weapons

(a) In General.—Whoever knowingly develops, produces, stockpiles, transfers, acquires, retains, or possesses any biological agent, toxin, or delivery system for use as a weapon, or knowingly assists a foreign state or any organization to do so, or attempts, threatens, or conspires to do the same, shall be fined under this title or imprisoned for life or any term of years, or both. There is extraterritorial Federal jurisdiction over an offense under this section committed by or against a national of the United States.

(b) Additional Offense.—Whoever knowingly possesses any biological agent, toxin, or delivery system of a type or in a quantity that, under the circumstances, is not reasonably justified by a prophylactic, protective, bona fide research, or other peaceful purpose, shall be fined under this title, imprisoned not more than 10 years, or both. In this subsection, the terms "biological agent" and "toxin" do not encompass any biological agent or toxin that is in its naturally occurring environment, if the biological agent or toxin has not been cultivated, collected, or otherwise extracted from its natural source.

(c) Definition.—For purposes of this section, the term "for use as a weapon" includes the development, production, transfer, acquisition, retention, or possession of any biological agent, toxin, or delivery system for other than prophylactic, protective, bona fide research, or other peaceful purposes.

(Added Pub. L. 101–298, §3(a), May 22, 1990, 104 Stat. 201; amended Pub. L. 104–132, title V, §511(b)(1), Apr. 24, 1996, 110 Stat. 1284; Pub. L. 107–56, title VIII, §817(1), Oct. 26, 2001, 115 Stat. 385; Pub. L. 107–188, title II, §231(c)(1), June 12, 2002, 116 Stat. 661.)

On April 1, 2021, an article written by US Army Reserve Colonel Lawrence Sellin (Ret.) discusses the connections[3] between Drs. Ralph Baric, Shi Zhengli-Li, Fang Li, and others, including Dr. Shibo Jiang. All are reportedly linked through Gain-of-Function research, US universities, and NIH and NIAID funding for millions of dollars.[4]

The previous chapters have provided detailed information showing the paper and money trails of those involved. The question now is, why would the US federal government, including NIAID, NIH, and the Department of Defense, become involved in the development of a bioweapon that violates the Biological Weapons Convention treaty, the Nuremberg Code, and the International Covenant on Civil and Political Rights (ICCPR) treaty? Why would the Chinese Communist Party (CCP) intentionally release SARS-CoV-2 in the wet market of Wuhan?

To begin to answer these questions, I participated in an interview per the request of Dr. Li Meng Yan and Dr. Karladine Graves in April 2021.[5] What follows is the transcript of that meeting. As you read through this interview, I would advise that you take Dr. Yan at her word. Based upon the US Senate Permanent Subcommittee on Investigations report by Chairman Rob Portman and Ranking Member Tom Carper, the senators clearly believe there is a real intent for China to develop biological weapons—weapons we have helped pay for! Yet the follow-up report[6] appears to have been since removed. For what reasons, I wonder?!

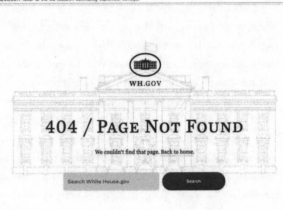

The Interview

"Lethal Deception," as published April 22, 2021 on Rumble "Torch of Freedom"[1]
Dr. Karladine Graves
Dr. Richard Fleming
Dr. Li Meng Yan

The following is a word-for-word transcription of the conversation featured on "Torch of Freedom."

Dr. Karladine Graves:
Welcome everyone—thank you very much for joining us. Tonight, we have a very honored, aah, physician—I guess you could say—Dr. Li Meng—from China, is here with us. And then Dr. Richard Fleming. Both of them are fabulous researchers—and they have the truth. And the truth is about the COVID-19 va . . . er, the COVID virus. So we are here tonight to help you to see what nefarious work has been done across this globe. And so welcome. We just want to thank you for joining us. So with that, I am going to ask Dr. Li Meng to introduce herself and tell us where she is from and also to tell us what type of work she has been doing.

Dr. Li Meng Yan:
Thank you, Dr. Karladine. Very happy to meet Dr. Richard too. Thank you for having me tonight. I am a doctor, and also a virologist, from China. And before I came to the US, I worked in University of Hong Kong (HK)—the WHO H5 Reference Lab—as a virologist working on the H1 universal vaccine development. So I am the first one who revealed that WHO has covered

up the whole things—the COVID-19 things—the Chinese Communist Party (CCP) in/and US, and [indistinguishable]. I started to video these things from the cover-up to the lab origin of the COVID-19 virus back to month of January on Chinese YouTube—anonymous, of course. My work is focusing, I mean, recently, it's focusing on how to help people understand the real origin of COVID-19. And also, when people realize it, I am happy to help people to figure out the possible solution and work with others— some will be doctors—and other people together—to find out the final solution. Thank you.

Dr. Karladine Graves:
Alright. Thank you. Dr. Fleming.

Dr. Richard Fleming:
Well, it's my pleasure to be here. And Dr. Li Meng, thank you for the invitation, and Karladine, for the invitation. This is an important thing you are doing for humanity, Dr. Li Meng. I am a physicist, nuclear cardiologist, with a law degree—attorney. I have fifty-two years' worth of research. A lot of that has gone into inflammation and various diseases like heart disease and cancer. I've also developed a method for measuring tissues changes. FMTVDM is a method that we've used during the last year in seven countries and twenty-three sites to look at SARS-CoV-2 and COVID patients for treatments. We've done a lot of work in the investigation on the origins of this virus, as well as the funding of it. And much of the information that I think Dr. Li Meng is going to tell you first hand . . . we've looked at papers and documents and can confirm what she's going to be telling you.

Dr. Karladine Graves:
That's wonderful. So in other words . . . actually, you two could work together. It sounds like this would be very advantageous for you both to continue on working together. So, this is truly a blessing. Thank you for actually asking, Dr. Li Meng, or Dr. Fleming. I think that you were right on. So I have a quick question for you. Do you think that the vaccine was actually being worked on even prior to COVID-19—actually the COVID virus being released?

Dr. Li Meng Yan:
Sorry, I didn't hear clearly.

Dr. Karladine Graves:
I'm sorry. Do you think that there was a vaccine that was being worked on prior to COVID-19 being released?

Dr. Li Meng Yan:
Aah. For the vaccine, I think you mean [indistinguishable]. Vaccine effective before they release SARS-CoV-2, right?

Dr. Karladine Graves:
That's what my question is. Were they already working on a vaccine before they released the virus?

Dr. Li Meng Yan:
Aah! So first I want to say this virus is already done as a known bioweapon. And according to the streakage—yes, they want also to have drugs and also vaccines—but as my first intelligence and my knowledge on CCP government, and their spin piece—and also based on the drill of [indistinguishable]. If you want to have the COVID-19 vaccine, I can tell you, they are trying to get the effective COVID-19 vaccine, but they don't have the effective vaccine. And especially when they release the virus—at that time—they don't have any vaccines they can use immediately and now they also don't have that. So, my opinion is—don't trust the vaccines developed from CCP government because in the history this government never have any vaccine successfully developed. And also, we, Chinese, all know, if we can afford the imported vaccine—I mean no matter what vaccines, we will choose the imported one rather than the made in China, the done-in-China vaccine. Because we also have many vaccine accidents before in our history.

Dr. Karladine Graves:
Go ahead, Dr. Fleming.

Dr. Richard Fleming:
Dr. Li Meng—question for you. The information that we have—the docs that show federal funding from the Department of Defense, Health and Human Services, NIH, NIAID, and a variety of US federal government sources—show that money was going from our federal government to Peter Dazsak at EcoHealth—who was then sending money then to Ralph Baric at the University of North Carolina and Zhengli at the Wuhan Institute of Virology (WIV). Do you have any info to confirm that that was kinda the

source of funding and that US funds—federal funds—were being used to help fund the development of this Gain of Function (GoF) bioweapon?

Dr. Li Meng Yan:
Aah, I think most people already have money evidence online, that, yes, US taxpayer money going towards the government funding and going to Mike Picacek [spelling unclear] and other people to the Chinese [indistinguishable] expansion [indistinguishable] like the WIV—and those funding was given to do at least a partial office [indistinguishable] project, and we cannot know that Dazsak is granted that this part is being done for the S protein, and that part is being done, like, for capture the virus. But we know that this is a—this is very important grant for the WIV, and WIV is really a very important lab in this Chinese unrestricted bioweapon project. It's not only one, but it is an important one. And also, [indistinguishable] the professors who get this grant from the US government, they were working for the GoF and also working on the bioweapon projects under the military single fusion project. So, what I can say is, follow this money, and finally you will see that US money did get involved into this project and later be used to hurt US, and also the world.

Dr. Richard Fleming:
Some other people have provided me information that says that Paris and Israel, and possibly the UK, were also involved in helping to fund and develop SARS-CoV-2. Do you know anything about that?

Dr. Li Meng Yan:
Aah, what I want to say is, this is a very big international network. And I can see not only one lab get involved. And you know China government—also including the labs in HK—and then you have a lot of international connections. Also, the money go around from these other countries to work with people in China or in Hong Kong. So in this huge network, I don't feel surprised if people can show that, yeah, maybe Israel's money, European money, goes into China. Because you also can see China's money goes to the European medical journals or scientists. So this is a mutual things' [indistinguishable]. Chinese government gets grants from other governments via some scientist and other people. Then they also gave the benefits back to them. So, if you say how many people get involved in this misinformation campaign [indistinguishable] from the beginning of the outbreak help Communist Party to cover up all the things I don't

think that people would be surprised that money out of US go to China has supported such project.

Dr. Richard Fleming:
Right. Some of the information that we have shows that this GoF research has been going on since right around 2002–2003. Do you know how far this goes back that they have been working on the GoF?

Dr. Li Meng Yan:
What I want to provide is . . . back to 2002, 2003—of course, at that time, I was just a fresh undergraduate [laughs]. I was not into that field. I was a clean-cut medical student the first year, the second year, at that time. But I worked with many people who were the top coronavirus expert. And, I think when people talk about 2002 to 2003, they definitely include information about at least one SARS outbreak. Because it happened in early 2003, right? So what I will say is, according to my knowledge, and also the evidence that I got from those experts—who really had the firsthand experience in SARS 1. Something that people can think about—it is no secret in the corona-virus research field, that is really interesting, that is, in SARS 1 outbreak, people are talking about the civet cat as the host, wild animal. And now, during SARS 2, people are looking for the wild host, and they didn't find the real host. But for civet cats in SARS 1. At that time, professor Guan Yee, in the University of Hong Kong, professor Manick Perris, and Dr. K. Y. Yin—these are all my ex-supervisors and the big professors working with. They are the ones who discover SARS 1 from civet cat. But civet cat car-rying SARS 1 is only found in some samples from a China market—a wet market in Guangzhou. So Professor Guan Yee got some notion that there may be the wild animal host samples in Guangzhou, and then they went to Guangzhou and [indistinguishable] help him to get some samples—like, ten to twenty—if I didn't remember wrong. And then he go back and found out, like half of them, were positive. Later, he went back to Guangzhou and got a second bunch of SARS 1 sample, and then they later confirmed that civet cat is host. But after that—but no one since—have found any civet cat with which carry the SARS 1 virus. And, also later, in 2015, there is a general who is a bioweapons expert who has been to Iraq for the bioweapon examination. His name is [indistinguishable], and he writes a textbook in PLA military schools, which get full way support from the PLA dogmatical staff and officers. SARS 1 is not nature origin. And, also, the title is about how to use an artificial virus to be the next generation of [indistinguishable]

weapons. I am not translating this book into English with my team. I want to show it to people in the US. So in this book, he actually writes the new strategy for the bioweapon. His idea is that SARS 1 is not from nature, and he thinks that SARS 1 evolution, and the SARS 1 that is artificial, and that later, somehow, disappeared. And, then his idea is to base on SARS 1—and the coronavirus—and people can or especially for the Chinese government. Because he is a PLA expert, they can have the new generation of the bioweapon using coronavirus—which can be different as a traditional bioweapon, like bacterias people know. So, they will have a different character. The different character, including first looks like zoonotic, looks like nature altering, as from animal. And also, the only thing you can see is history, evolution history—actually disobeys the nature of evolution history. But these things once the things can be found out the government can deny and also, the important thing they also mention that seafood market would be a good place to release it. So, if we go back to check the SARS 2, we will see SARS 2 actually perfectly matched their idea. And there are also other things inside like the bioweapon which can circulate [indistinguishable] while masking among the population [indistinguishable] human population and also the animal and environment [indistinguishable]. And the important thing is that they don't care about mortality that much. Because mortality is not the case. They are focusing on some bioweapon which is hidden, easy to be transmitted. And also Et Can Zhoun [indistinguishable] [the society?] economic, social disorder of the enemy's country. So, I think when people thing, see these things come out of from PLA bioweapon's expert's mouth for years, people will understand the nature of SARS 2 and can also think of SARS 1 whether it's from nature or not.

Dr. Karladine Graves:
I have a question. Some of the physicians I work with are reporting more and more that their patients are coming up positive for HIV. Some of them is after the vaccine. My question is—and I have seen a study out of India—last year—and it was probably last March—where supposedly four scientists has sequenced the virus, and in the COVID-19 vaccine there appeared to be four glycoprotein 120s that had actually came from the HIV virus. Do you know anything about that at all?

Dr. Li Meng Yan:
I think I have read that paper as you mention. I see people talking about this. For me, what I want to say about this, I am not a virologist in HIV

study, so I think this, I mean, of course this virus has combined ma[?]
things together. Except for the things I revealed in my [indistinguishabl[?]]
reports there should be other characters or evidence left. So I think thi[?]
should be left for the HIV experts to discuss. My idea is according to that
analyze first the settlement the point is the *shot*. So it can be something
maybe from the HIV or maybe they designed something else, and that its
sequence is in common. But for me, I don't make such judgment, and also
I think it is important to say that is what has function because as we know,
especially the S protein has been modified like 30 to 40 percent according
to the backbone [?] [indistinguishable], there should be a lot of secrets hidden
inside. Some maybe not meaningful. Some meaningful significance. So
these things are important for people to discuss, and what I want emphasis
is from the beginning, I want to tell people is the lab origin and also the
evidence of the lab origin in this virus and also is not from IPG 13 but from
the [indistinguishable] bat coronavirus.

It's because once people understand/realize the real backbone they will
go back to check how much difference exactly from nature bat coronavirus
to this SARS 2. And they will focus on the difference between the backbone
and SARS 2. The difference actually for the whole virus is over 10 percent,
not just 4 percent as RaTG13 mentioned. If you only focus on 4 percent, it
means at least 6 percent or more difference will be ignored. Especially for
this SARS 2, we see the sig effect happen on the human ACE E2 receptor
with the RBD and also furin cleavage site where the virus enter to the cell.
But we should also know that when we see a lot of communications [possibly
said commutations] that cannot be explained and is higher than SARS
1 and other coronavirus and also we see the different character, unusual
character are all combined into SARS 2 to give the harmful effect to people.
We really need focus; there is a much/most secret that happen in the next
6 percent of the difference. So whether they learn from the HIV or they
are from hantavirus, we can see something in common from even YF virus
and also Ebola and something so that works the other scientists to dig, and
they prove their findings in their labs, so once people are allowed to talking
about lab origin encouraged to do this [indistinguishable] can help them to
support their work in lab origin study. I am sure more and more doctors will
have very good outcomes to help us understand the virus.

Dr. Richard Fleming:

Yes, I think, and you mentioned, the PRRA or the furin cleavage site that
isn't present in any other virus that exists on the planet. But clearly the

genetics show there is a PRRA insert on the spike protein for SARS-CoV-2, which shows, I believe, human intent and GoF.

Dr. Li Meng Yan:
Yes. PRRA [indistinguishable] cleavage site and, of course, furin cleavage site—also happened in Ebola, [indistinguishable] high passaging in Florida virus, even in hantavirus, and also MERS. But first they are not a known HIV B beta coronavirus—and also, in this site, we actually see this is something artificial inserted. I provide the genome sequence—that evidence— and who have died, people who have such experience in reference in my first Yan report. I think people can verify by themselves and this PRRA—we have seen a lot papers have done before—to show like—if you insert it into the low passaging influenza virus it will become a high passaging one, and if you remove it from SARS it will de-tenure it—make it become a life-attentive virus. So this is a functional segment which is not confirmed by nature, recombination, or evolution. But there is also here as in FAUL—the site inside—which can help people to monitor whether this furin cleavage site get lost during experiment. So, I really think, first, this a smoking-gun-level evidence to show that this is lab modification and GoF modification. And, also, they have done it in a very deliberate way, which can have both cleavage site function and also [indistinguishable] function. So, they really care about this function. They don't want to lose it during [indistinguishable] A7 [indistinguishable] experiment.

Dr. Richard Fleming:
I think it's really interesting that the patent for furin cleavage protease enzymes is owned by the US.

Dr. Li Meng Yan:
·Pattern of what? Aah, I'm sorry?

Dr. Richard Fleming:
The pattern for the [furin cleavage protease enzymes] is owned by the US, and the federal government has patent rights to it.

Dr. Li Meng Yan:
Patent belongs to whom it is important, but it is not the real important thing when people use it. According to what Chinese government thinks, whatever you have I can get it. I can steal.

Dr. Richard Fleming:
Right.

Dr. Li Meng Yan:
I don't want to humiliate the Chinese scientists—I am sure many Chinese scientists—working with me—they are very honest and don't do such things. But there are always some people. You know when they got . . . you know . . . Chinese government uses money and big titles—and so these things to attract them; they will do this, and this is something that kinda an open secret in the Chinese scientific world. So these things with the US, and then Chinese research, Chinese scientists bring it back—even US scientists bring these other country scientists, bring these techniques to China. This is common. So pay attention to that some people may ask if this is designed in the US. But what I want to emphasize is, the backbone of this SARS 2, it comes from China PLA Chinese army-owned, this owned unit, the unique bat coronavirus they say Chinese government they say forty-five or accident twenty-one, is China government is the one leading the cover-up and spreading the misinformation—don't allow people to check or to do more investigation—and even cannot talk about it—censor these things. So we can clearly see who is the one making.

Dr. Richard Fleming:
Perfect.

Dr. Karladine Graves:
So the bottom line is this. I am just going to ask to make it very clear for those that are going to be listening to this, then: this virus, that we are dealing with right now, is *not* something that happens in nature, and it appears that this is a bio-engineered effort—and, that it was an international effort—and not just necessarily one or two—but probably from this country, and the UK, as Dr. Fleming was saying, and many others. Am I correct in saying that?

Dr. Li Meng Yan:
I think from designing to equip—of course—this is a project, directed plan, by the CCP government, and the biggest job [indistinguishable] behind is Chinese military medical academy. We can see their shadow behind those work. And, also, there are a lot of civil labs got involved, like WIV, and even there are many important experience come from my previous lab—University

of HK—a WHO lab—and, beside these things, there are a lot of international scientists donated inside, but these international scientists, they may not know the real things that got involved, because the CCP won't trust anyone, especially when there is a foreigner from foreign country which is not that easy to be controlled. But they know how to use like, money, or scientific, or use paper, use promotion opportunities—all these things to influence and then cover it up. And also the money—as we discussed before—from different countries has payers—goes into China because they feel China is providing some environment to give them good outcome. But actually, this money was secretly being used for this kind of bad purpose, and also, somehow, they managed to get rid of the international surveillance. And meanwhile, those medical journals, *The Cell*, *Nature*, [indistinguishable], *Lancet*, *New England*, they also got very well collaboration with the CCP because Chinese government gave a lot of money to help them develop—and, also, there are a lot of people who can get a good exchange of maybe other part-time accounts in China. So these journals also help the CCP in covering up and also spreading misinformation and doing the censorship.

So this is long term—after the case there came a long-term streakage [strategy?] in CCP, and during this time, they did make a big international—I mean, *huge* international network involving the important scientists, the important journals, important organization like WHO, [indistinguishable] NIH [indistinguishable], and all this, even media, together. That's why, when it happened, most of people—even scientists —fall into their pit—that this is from nature or this is something that we cannot treat as how we call it a novel vaccine. All these things actually are made up to help the Chinese government achieve their evil goal.

Dr. Karladine Graves:
Well, I have been told that the editors of many of these journals have received quite a bit of money, that there was money exchanged for articles that—certainly not only China—but big pharmaceuticals also—are trying to slant that info. When I was—I'm older—so when I went to med school after I got out, the *New England Journal of Medicine*, and so on, was kind of the mainstay of us knowing what was up to date. So is what you're saying that these journals are not really reliable for truth?

Dr. Li Meng Yan:
Yes, what I want to say is, first, the journal, actually—itself—cannot distinguish the real information and the misinformation, so they rely on the

reviewer. And the reviewer, if they have good, very good, connection with the CCP, or if they are influenced by the top biologists or scientists which is influenced by the CCP, this will make them have the wrong decision and idea. What I can say is just talking about [indistinguishable] 13. I have many examples happen around me before that I know how involve even the editor of *Nature* that showcased his attitude towards my ex-boss—I don't want to talk about that now, but I can show you another example which is ITJ 13 [indistinguishable] virus actually. Many scientists are questioning the existence of the virus. Whether it is a real virus and because there are a lot of problems. I also show in my secondary project, and [indistinguishable] many other scientists think there are problems and, at least, they need Dr. Zhingli or other people to explain it. Or, maybe *Nature* journal can do an investigation as to whether they should withdraw it. I am one of the people who have helped people to write an email asked *Nature* to give a response to this. I think this was last June or July. My name was not on this, but I helped some other people also write such letter. And I know there was, at least, several other letters sent to *Nature*, but none of them as I know gathered response. And, still now, you say also more and more people asked the questions ITJ 13, but *Nature* still kept on publishing the papers based it IRTJ 13 and don't care about this paper's evidence and whether it is real well or not. So this is a very good example for the world to see. And also, another thing is, according to the exposed email between Pete Dazsak, and also many, many top scientists in the world, we can see how they work together to write that famous *Lancet* [indistinguishable] statement from the end of last January and published last February in *Lancet* to praise CCP in anti-COVID-19—and also insist that nature origin of SARS-CoV-2, although they don't have any evidence. And, also, at the same time, this meets the lab origins that this is definitely a conspiracy. I am sure it makes me want to ask those people, "How are you so confident to write such statements?" At least the [indistinguishable] didn't say their evidence. Until now we only know that they tried—if it happened *or* if something happened that may be or that can be. Right? We didn't say anything else. No solid evidence. And then there are the other ones who are ignoring the evidence of lab origins and dismiss people who are talking about lab origin GoF of COVID-19 virus.

Dr. Richard Fleming:

Yes. *Conspiracy* is the beautiful term they like to use in social media—which is the idea that there must be some mistake about that, forgetting the fact that conspiracy has a real meaning. It means more than one person getting together to do something nefarious that they shouldn't be doing. So, if there is a conspiracy, it is a real phenomenon of more than one person getting together to do this harmful thing. And the beauty of it is that they have so confused people on the idea that this is somehow naturally occurring when there is no way in the world it could be by looking at the genetic code. And you have the general public around the world crying out for the suppression of the truth and reinforcement of the misinformation—which is probably exactly what the CCP is looking for.

Dr. Li Meng Yan:
When we see the evidence, we can always see two arms of possibility—one is from nature, one is from lab. And, then, we can see the evidence to compare which possibility is more reliable. And, then, we see until now we wait for one year we only see that fabricated data or series come out from the nature original series. They told us to span out one thousand years waiting for maybe the real ancestor of SARS 2. Or maybe we need to chase the bat, I mean, for our next life even to find out some unknown bat coronavirus. On the other side, there are a lot of smoking guns left in the SARS-CoV-2. And also, in my series [indistinguishable] report, I provide who has done this, who is good at it, and who enjoys doing that. So if you compare the two sides, I think many people with common sense and knowledge can get their own conclusion.

So, back to the conspiracy—it's very funny. There are two words I want to mention in the SARS-CoV-2 pandemic. One is conspiracy. The other is politics. So once those scientists working with China government—and they try to tell people it comes from nature—they just charge anyone else not on their side as someone has a political opinion which want to spread the conspiracy. But what I want to say is, first, this is not conspiracy because we already talk about the evidence. We see the evidence is more solid in the lab-origin side. And we encourage people to talk about it—and even nature-origin people can come to debate with us. At least for me, I tell people open debate is always welcome, and I list as a scientist from CCP who have done such things, who are experts in those fields, and even those people from HK and the US—all these people, I welcome them to have open discussion with me in the right style, influential media (they can choose the media)—I don't mind—we just present our evidence. Right? If you have more evidence, I respect it, and I will welcome that side to do more evidence to present people some "chunks" to get understand of the virus.

And, the other one about politics—people started talking about if you mention China government or CCP, that means it is politics. *No!* It's not politics. I mean, it doesn't mean that party or government is equal to politics. At least, for me, here, for the lab origin—I will tell—Zhi Zhengli is the one claimed to have ITJ 13. So I will also tell you that SARS-CoV-2 is hidden and made by the CCP because this is the name of the group of the people that have done that. This is just like I am telling the officer. What else word I can use? Right? There is always name it party or government [indistinguishable] because of the present view of that organization?! I cannot just say Chinese, because I am also Chinese. Not every Chinese person will do such bad things. Right? And also everyone got involved, and this is not politics; this a real thing happened to us involved the global health, our [indistinguishable] and our next generation—even animal health. Right? So don't just judge that as conspiracy or politics unless you are very politic sensitive population or unless you think your life, your health, is only something simple as the politics issue.

Dr. Richard Fleming:
Yes. That is perfectly said. I think reality is the science of looking at this virus tells us where it came from, what we need to be doing about it, and how we need to be addressing it globally on the planet and to quit looking at people as Chinese or American, given that we funded so much of this or anybody else. It is to have an open, honest debate and discussion about it. A failure to be able to do this is very telling that you don't have much evidence of your own to stand on.

Dr. Karladine Graves:
Can we talk just a little bit about—everyone wants to mask. Any thoughts about how small this virus is and it goes through masks? Do either of you have any comments on this?

Dr. Li Meng Yan:
Yes. OK. Thank you. I have some thoughts about masks. First thing: Masks is not universal. I don't think it is healthy to wear masks all day long—especially when you are exercising. It is not good for your breathing. *Right?* Also I don't support that kind of wearing masks for kids for years; some people try to support mask policy. I don't think it's very useful for kids to wear growing up masks all the time. It's not good for some development. There is some study that shows that kids need to develop their face-recognizing function and also other social schemes, and masks maybe can weaken this

function development. But the thing is, my idea is, in the SARS-2 pandemic, some masks can be helpful in certain situation. So yes, the virus particle is very little. It—from the size—it can go through even the N95 mask. But we know that this is the virus which can be attached to the droplet—air drop—and the droplet can go through the airborne way. The mask can stop this kind of droplet on the surface. Surgical masks can do some. And also N95 mask is a little better than surgical mask.

So once this air drop and droplet stop on the surface and if you know how to wear the mask in the proper way, this does give you some possibility that the virus will not go into your mouth or touch you get infected. And this is something having shown from some outcome. I think we still encourage more studies because I see people questioning whether the data is solid. But one paper is from my previous lab in HK; that group people showed in some situations surgical masks and N95 can prevent somewhere between 20 to 40 percent of the infection in that situation. And also, another group from Professor Yugi Kawaka—he is the big influenza virologist—and he also issued the model to mimic if one person is coughing in front of you and in a short distant 1 meter and if the viral concentration is very high, then in his study, that cotton masks may prove 70 percent effective if I remember right, and also surgical masks can be like 20 to 30 percent prevention, and N95 is higher. But we know, these are all under the experimental environment, so we still know there are limitations. I encourage more people to do study of this. Before that, I think, maybe, for example, if you know how to wear the mask in the proper way—so wear the N95 in a very crowded setting—in a protest or other this kind of situation—with people very close—it can maybe help you to reduce the chance to get infection. But if you don't know how to wear a mask properly, like you touch the surface and then touch your face, and then you wear it and remove it and wear it again—in a random way—I don't think that will be helpful.

Dr. Karladine Graves:
Well, I've noticed when you go to restaurants, they usually take it off and put it on the table.
[Laughing]

Dr. Li Meng Yan:
That's very interesting. You stand up, you wear it, and you sit down, and you can take it off. And you eat in that way. I don't think in that way will be very helpful.

Dr. Richard Fleming:

Yeah. And I always tell people whether a mask is beneficial or not depends on what type of mask you are wearing and where you are at. If you are in a hospital setting or in an area where there is a high concentration of people with SARS-CoV-2, and there is a great chance of it being spread, wearing a mask appropriately will reduce the potential transmission. But I think if you are not around people that are coughing or sneezing or around a lot of people that are infected, then I think there is very little evidence to support the wearing of the masks. This entire concept of sending elementary school and secondary kids to school and wearing masks and claiming that there is evidence that protects them. That evidence is not there. There is a lot of misinformation out there, and none of it supports the wearing of masks by kids in secondary school systems. None of it supports, I think, from what I have seen, the wearing of it in the general population because unless people are contagious, and you are around them in close proximity, the spread is so minimal that it is unconscionable to be wearing the masks. And there are problems with social barriers and a number of other problems coming from that. But if you are in a hospital setting and you are around patients with SARS-CoV-2 or COVID-19—if they develop the disease—now it becomes an intelligent thing to actually do. So the mask—like so many things—has become like so many other things—an either/or debate—as opposed to instead of what's the science behind when is it right and when it's not. And that's where we need to be focusing.

Another thing I want to discuss are the vaccines. Because recognizing that the vaccines are nothing but the genetic codes of the spike protein and recognizing that the spike protein is manmade GoF. What the vaccines are, are an intro into the human body of something that is not naturally occurring, that are the very thing that people made that shouldn't be going into human bodies—and certainly, not being encoded for our bodies to make massive quantities of. The vaccines, Pfizer and Moderna, have 13.1 billion mRNAs per administration. The Jansen (or J & J) has 50 billion. And, when you consider the fact, from my perspective, as I am now look- ing at the data, there are two things really going on in the world of vac- cines. One is a delivery mechanism, and one is, "Why would they want to do that?" Well, inserting something that is man-made into people instead of addressing the fact that it's man-made and treating it with appropriate medications (and doing the right thing), is tantamount to chaos. And it's running amuck. So, then you have to ask why they would want to be able to do these vaccines? And this provides you with the opportunity to do things to people that they would not normally allow you to do—which is to stick things into their bodies. And when you consider the fact that the very people who have been doing the funding on the US side—people like Bill Gates, the Leona Helmsley Foundation, and a group of people, that to be very blunt, are criminal pedophile organizations providing money, and you notice they are also funding CRISPR tech, and then you listen to their discussion of going in with CRISPR. . . . The limitation of CRISPR tech was that it did not have a delivery mechanism. And what these vaccines have done is answered the delivery mechanism problem. I think it's very interesting that this whole thing with GoF and producing something as a bioweapon has not just produced a bioweapon to take down countries and economies by putting everyone into this fear and separation mode, but its provided the next opportunity for these same people, funding all this, to develop a vaccine mechanism now with CRIPSR tech to do . . . I don't know what they are planning to do with that. They are going to have to answer for that, but none of it is a good scientific or positive thing for human beings.

Dr. Karladine Graves:
Do you want to comment on that?

Dr. Li Meng Yan:
I do have my concern about the vaccine now. And the first thing is, I keep telling people there are no real effective vaccines against the pandemic. So there are some reasons, very simple for people can understand. So first thing is—this virus SARS-CoV-2 is basically the big version, the enhanced version of SARS 1. And we never have SARS 1 vaccine. I am not antivaccine. I work on universal influenza vaccine. I have my patent on Pandy. I just know how to develop vaccines in the proper way. Right?! Try in proper way. So this SARS-CoV-2, like SARS 1—we don't have vaccine because it side effects and contains like other allergy or antibody dependent enhancement (ADE). And also we don't have a good universal influenza vaccine [indistinguishable] it's because of the quick mutation. So now SARS comes, and the quick, and it also has the mutation in the circulation, and it also has side effects of SARS 1. So how can people quickly overcome these issues in several months? And, also, we know that SARS 2 actually also has a lot of modifications—as Dr. F also mentioned. It's a bioweapon. I already showed that it's an unrestricted bioweapon, so there are also many hidden functions [indistinguishable] transmission issue.

So, at least now, you see we are using most appropriately, we are using the S protein equipped as our adenovirus or MRA factors and delivered to our body. I don't judge the technique because I didn't see a lot of technique data released by these MRA companies. So we need to examine this when it is openly released—more released data—and we can know more. But just talk about S protein. That whether there is hidden function inside, we don't know. But we do see that people got infected and get more complications like we just mentioned. So at this time it is just delivered as protein to our body. We don't know whether it will be some other worse effect, which is even ignored or may not come out in the short term, but in the chronic style later in our bodies. Or whether it will induce some problem that can be treated by some other factor when we get vulnerable. We don't know that. We just know that we still need more data, animal data, original data, and also small human child data. This needs to be done under very strict surveillance and also a lot of people—scientists—should check the data carefully and open discuss it. We don't know that. We just see that the vaccine is given to people; even when people have other baseline problems. Even when they are old. I don't know, for example, in China they give some in HK for the inactive or other type of vaccine—the single vaccine—from that company to the senior age group. I'm not sure if it is inactive or recommended—anyway they give some to a senior age group over sixty years. That is a special group. In vaccine development, you know that senior people have lower immunity—immune response—so whether the vaccine will work for them has to be done in a specific this age of population for small trial. And also, because in this age group—they usually have diabetes or hypertension or other problems. We have to think whether this combination will affect this vaccine.

But now it seems it just come into human and then people see the results. And we even didn't see the very clear result although the vaccine has been given for several months. Right? So now, I really feel it is hurry to get the vaccine. And we do encourage the pharmacy to generate more data to show people—for the scientific world—to discuss whether we could improve and do it better. If not, I feel we are some animal model for the real animals' vaccine. Maybe later mouse will have some very safe COVID-19 vaccine because we gave them enough data.

And also, meanwhile, we have to look into the prophylaxis drugs or early treatment drugs—so cheap, long-term use, and will prove to be safe like drugs hydroxycholorquine, ivermectin, or other things—that are cocktail recipients—cocktail protocols—and a lot based on previous treatment using these drugs. And these drugs can do many things to stop the spreading of the virus. It's not magic, but it is worth it to be applied.

Dr. Richard Fleming:
Right. You know we've published papers showing treatments that actually work 99.83 percent of the time—as opposed to everybody throwing their hands up and saying there is no treatment. You know one of the other things about the spike protein that we haven't touched on yet is the fact that that there is a prion-like domain at the receptor binding site of the spike protein. And the animal models that I've seen—and the humanized mice models—and the rhesus macaque models—both show neurologic damage as a result of the spike protein crossing the blood-brain barrier. And, so, in the humanized mice models, they are actually showing spongiform encephalopathy with 95 percent of the animals dying within two weeks (which is mad cow disease for those of the audience that don't speak medicine). And then, in the rhesus macaque models, they are showing lewy bodies and microglia and other inflammatory cells in the brains of these rhesus macaque—also in about five to six weeks. So, there is clear data doing the scientific method with animal models in the investigation of a virus—which is the way we should be investigating this virus and the vaccines—that there neurologic long-term sequelae that's coming up as a result of these spike proteins and there are some papers that are showing up now that the vaccines themselves are promoting this same potential for neurologic damage. Dr. Li Meng, I don't know what is going through most peoples' minds scientifically or medically, when everybody is ignoring the scientific model and method that we have used for many, many decades on how to appropriately do this sort of thing? But, you know, you make all sorts of very good points for the importance about doing this methodically and intelligently to get answers, so we are doing the right thing for people responding to this bioweapon.

Dr. Karladine Graves:
I was just going to say that today I received a call, that in my neighboring state over here in Kansas, that I had two patients that I was taking care of that did get COVID-19, and I was treating with hydroxychloroquine and so on. This was maybe two months ago. And they did well and recovered quite nicely. However, they went on and got the vaccine. And after they got the vaccine, they became very ill. And then, I treated them again, just as I would a COVID-19 patient. They went on to report this to the Health

Department that actually let them know, from their tracing department (that they were referred to), that 90 percent of those that they had vaccinated at the Health Department, in that particular [indistinguishable], now were coming down with COVID-19.

Dr. Li Meng Yan:
Ninety percent?

Dr. Karladine Graves:
Ninety percent is what they said. Yes, ma'am. I even called back. Because I thought I don't want to say this if this is not what they said. But they said that 90 percent of those that they had given the vaccine to that they had come down with COVID.

Dr. Li Meng Yan:
After how long was it when they got vaccine?

Dr. Karladine Graves:
That was just within a few weeks. I also have a gentleman—I am helping the family—he was just fine—he had no health issues. And after he received his two injections then he began hallucinating. And he would run out into the yard and think there was the police taking his son away and trying to fight these imaginary people that he was hallucinating about, and the family took him to the hospital, and they said he has a very rapid onset dementia. Well, I think it is just exactly what Dr. F said. I think it was actually the frontal temporal lobe, the problem that happens when the brain actually turns into like a sponge. And I think he probably actually has something of that nature.

Dr. Li Meng Yan:
May I ask something? They do have one COVID-19 before, and get treated, and they recovered, right?

Dr. Karladine Graves:
That is correct.

Dr. Li Meng Yan:
So, they should have the antibodies, I mean, at least 80 percent of the time they should have antibodies. They are lasting in their bodies. And then

they—first thing—why do they still need to get a vaccine at this time if they still have the antibodies? Nature offering antibody. The second thing is—besides other possibilities, let me say, next time catch the pathogen—at least part of the pathogen—from coronavirus and get some of the worst effect which is not by the Health Department as COVID-19 symptoms. And what I want to ask is, is there anything related to the antibody have before—is this kind of antibody intense dependence enhancement from COVID-19?

Dr. Karladine Graves:
Um hmm. Exactly. Are both of you concerned about the antibody dependent enhancement (ADE)?

Dr. Richard Fleming:
Absolutely! The Osaka, Japan, paper, that was published well back in 2020, showed that this spike protein has antibodies that form not only to the receptor binding domain but to the end terminal. And when those antibodies form to the end terminal, it causes a conformational change in the spike protein, opening up the regional binding domain—increasing the infectivity of the spike protein. This is not the type of ADE we have seen before. This is a different type of ADE. And it doesn't matter—in fact, some of the patients in the hospital that have not done well, even though they have antibodies, when they look at them they have more antibodies to the end terminal domain. If you throw a spike protein into somebody's body, they are going to make both types, and it's just a matter of which one they are making more of as to what the outcomes are. And that end terminal domain is present in those spike proteins, and that gene sequence that the spike protein are being made. And this tells us also that we are dealing with something that has not been seen before. Because we don't have that type of problem of another type of antibody forming to an end terminal domain enhancing the infectivity of the spike protein. This hasn't been seen with other types of ADE phenomenon. So yes. The fact that someone gets ill from SARS-CoV-2 forms the antibodies, recovers. All of that plays into the question as to whether there are end terminal domain antibodies floating around and whether the vaccine is introducing something to promote more of that problem. You know just making antibodies is not always a good thing. Strep pharyngitis or strep throat, the reason why we, as physicians—particularly cardiologists—treat you, is because we don't want you making antibodies, because the antibodies to strep pneumonia—the antigens to

which—look an awful lot like your mitral and aortic valve, which causes rheumatic heart disease. So just because you can make an antibody doesn't necessarily mean it's a good thing. Making the wrong type of antibody can enhance in this type of infectious agent that's man-made. All of this just speaks to a lack of scientific, fundamental knowledge in the people that are running the paradigm on this socially.

Dr. Li Meng Yan:

I am not a neurologist; I just have the medical knowledge about neurological disease, but what I have pondered in my third report, and also in my first, and I kept using it as a smoking gun—is the envelop protein or E protein. In SARS-CoV-2 it is 100 percent identical [indistinguishable] as the backbone of the Gaoshan bat coronavirus. First, this is evidence that it comes from the Gaoshan bat coronavirus—which is, somehow, conveniently capped into SARS-CoV-2. Because if it is going rough, the species that kind of host changing and jump from bat to animal to animal to human—definitely we will see the change because we already observed the change during the early pandemic in human. And second thing is, why do they keep it? Because this is a smoking gun. And I write this problem from last year 19th of January, with YouTube. China government quickly get response and later they even lock up because they know someone release the real information about this bioweapon. But why until now? No scientist there to touch this E protein issue to argue with me. Even Zhengli, and their Chinese Military Academy, they have developed a lot of novel, fabricated, zoonotic, virus—including bats or from pangolins—which all have the identical E protein in those fabricated sequence. What do they want to hide? Then, let's back to check E protein's function. Yes. It's not clearly investigated. But we know it's important for virus and modification and for some other important parts in the coronavirus. But it also have another function. What is discovered actually in my ex-lab (University of HK), is the lab that got involved to discover this, is E protein can help the virus maintain the new toxicity. I don't mean that this is some maybe smoking gun. It still need people to do more study transmission problem. But I also want to tell people, "Why do they choose Gaoshan bat coronavirus—they say forty-five or they accept twenty-one? I want to tell people some information—back to 2009 to 2014, there is big national grant conducted by the China cities that have Charles Bugal. He encouraged the people in the multilab region to finish this project by capturing and identifying the novel zoonotic virus all over China. Including coronavirus, dengue, or Zika or hantavirus—all this—and for this—all the virus. There is one thing is interesting in this five year project—every year—he wanted to have people find two to three types of the novel virus with the capacity to impact the brain—neural toxicity. Why? Every year, two to three if they can complete this goal. That means ten to fifteen novel virus will be found during five years. But later, when I checked the data, I didn't see at least so many coronavirus were found with neurotoxicity function. But later, from 2015 to 2017, so Dr. Guan Chan Ching, from the 3rd Military Medical University, conducted the project in the Cape, capturing the zoonotic virus—and then, from the bat virus, he found ZC45 and ZXC21 [indistinguishable], so he published the paper showing something unusual. Because this is a bat coronavirus, and then they just checked whether this can infect the suckling bat, and then they found in the suckling bat brain, information. Very significant information. So for me, I am doing the research with this, and I am checking on other things, but use suckling rat to do these thing and present when you just identify a novel virus. And then later, there are no other functioning downstream publications, this is something very weird. Whether it is a one trip some standard and then because E protein can maintain the neurotoxicity, so they wanted the GoF enhancing the neurotoxicity, they want to keep the E protein—at least—for safety. I think this is a question worthy of the scientists for more investigation. Especially when we see there are a third of people from the report lately that have neurologic disorder—including the information or maybe the emotional change. We do have to focus on this thing and see if there is something that comes back [indistinguishable].

Dr. Karladine Graves:
Do either of you see this as a national security issue? Because we are giving this to our first responders, to our military, our police. Do you see it as a national security issue?

Dr. Li Meng Yan:
I think we need more data to check it. Because, at least now, we see the adverse effects resulting and they published the data is not that high—but that is just in a short period for a short distance first. Short period. Just after we start the vaccination for two or three months, right? So we don't know where there will be something that comes out later. For example, I see some reports online that say some women's cycles show changed, and then when they reported it clinical—they get a response that this is not included as part of the worst effects. So whether this kind of unusual adverse effect or

included in this kind of data is also very important. And also, yes, I think people, I mean government, should treat this very seriously. And we don't say the vaccine should be 100 percent safety. Of course, if the vaccine should be 100 percent safety for individuals. But when we use the massive vaccination, we should guarantee that most of the people will be in a healthy condition. Especially now, with the doctors, nurses, and soldiers, all the important people, they get vaccines. Imagine! If something happened!?! How would they protect the country, and how would they treat the patients? And you know when we get into mess last year—it is not because of the mortality—it is because of the disorder in hospitals or it is because of the sudden pandemic. So we should get avoid all these things of sudden mess-up, and all these things should be noted by the government.

Dr. Richard Fleming:
I would echo that. I think that at this point in time, there is absolutely no reason for this vaccine to be given to anybody—any of these vaccines. I think that we don't know what they are doing to people. Their data —daily or weekly—from the VAERS that's reporting on it—only shows more and more harm to people and more and more deaths. The EUA documents show—if you actually run the numbers—show nothing statistically significant about a reduction in the numbers of COVID or reductions in the deaths. So we are using experimental drugs—pan vaccinating the entire country—when we have drugs that can actually treat the infection and the disease when it's there. And we have no idea what the ramifications of these vaccines are. We are going to find out. I mean everybody is either part of the experimental or the control group at this point in time, like it or not.

Dr. Karladine Graves:
I'll be part of the control group!

Dr. Richard Fleming:
Your best chance of not coming down with SARS-CoV-2 or COVID is to do one of three things:

1. Improve your overall health and reduce the comorbidities that increase your risk for having a bad outcome if you get infected.
2. Actually be treated by a physician with medications that we know treat the infection or the disease.

3. Join the control group in one of these vaccine trials, because other than the people in South Africa, people aren't dying from COVID-19 in these COVID trials—if they are on the No Vaccine, in contrast to more than 2,600 who have now died following one of these three vaccines.

The more this hits the healthy and the young, the worse it is. It's clearly not good to hit the older people and people with disease. For the life of me, I cannot fathom why anyone would be excited about vaccinating our children, particularly down to age two or three, with a vaccine that's an experimental drug. And if it hits our military, and it hits our police, and it hits our frontline people, if it hits the doctors and nurses, it becomes a crisis for another means. If it hits the general population and causes damage, it is a crisis for the reason of causing harm to the general population. But there is nothing good that comes out of the way that we are approaching this right now: Ignoring the fact that this is a bioweapon and man-made. Ignoring the fact that there are medications that treat it. Ignoring the fact that we rushed to put together vaccines that haven't been proven to reduce the instance statistically of either coming down with COVID-19 or dying. All of that just raises a serious question of what happened to the human race and the intelligence. And if the goal was to cause chaos and panic, it's been successful.

Dr. Karladine Graves:
Yes, it has. Do either of you think that those individuals who received the vaccine—if they are actually shedding some virus?

Dr. Richard Fleming:
My response to that is—I have reviewed papers that have not been accepted for publication due to flaws or errors in methodology, studies that looked at sputum, stool, blood, and urine samples over a protracted period of time from people that got infected. And fortunately, the methodology that was done was done in such a poor manner that they couldn't guarantee the location of where the people were getting infected. So the answer is, I don't know how much shedding there is—if there's shedding going on. We don't have the data. I don't know if people who have had the vaccination are shedding and are infectious to others. We don't have the data. We do know—from Moderna—that when lipid nanoparticles—injections—are made into muscle from the influenza studies that were done with lipid nanoparticles that the vaccine does not stay in the site of the muscle. In the animal models

that they actually published their data on a few years ago—back in 2017, I believe—the lipid nanoparticles, and the influenza virus that was connected with it, showed up in the brain, the bone marrow, the liver, the spleen, every organ in the animal. So to think that we are injecting these vaccines into muscles and they are staying there is ignoring the science that was published by Moderna—one of the three companies!

Dr. Li Meng Yan:
The virus itself is very high contagious, and it can be easily transmitted from person to person. And when person get vaccination—it doesn't mean he cannot get the virus at least attached to himself. So he is still has a chance once the person has contacted a high concentration of the virus. And I think—imagine the person—any type of even the surface which when the highest concentration of the virus is attached—and other people attach this surface—will have the chance to get infected. And their vaccination doesn't mean that this surface won't have the highest concentration of virus attached. And, so in this way, I cannot say when you get vaccinated and the people can touch you very safely and even that vaccine can protect you. For this character of SARS-CoV-2, I still think this is a potential risk for healthy people to—to contact very closely—unless, the people who get vaccinated also wash their hands, take care of themselves, and I still think that practicing the safety when people get infected [indistinguishable] prophylaxis [indistinguishable] and that is the real way so that drugs can protect the virus from various mechanisms. Basically, it is like eliminating the pull of the virus. This is the fundamental way to remove the virus from our life. If I get vaccine, I do not see this as a cure from people's contacting.

Dr. Karladine Graves:
Well, we have gone over an hour. [some small talk] Dr. Li Meng, aren't you taking a risk? You're kind of in hiding aren't you?

Dr. Li Meng Yan:
Yes. Kind of hiding some, in the east of the US. As I said, I am the one to do these things. Because I am one actually of the first scientists who gets involved into the investigation of SARS-CoV-2 back to December 31, 2019. And later, I revealed the things because of the cover-up and the delay from the CCP. So I revealed it anonymously through a Chinese YouTube [indistinguishable] when I was in HK to give the warning to the world. And the one thing I can tell you, there are five parts which are all verified

later—include at that time it is nineteenth of January, 2020, and I tell people there are rarely human-to-human transmission like this and the virus can be highly mutant and if it's not, the Chinese government, and also the WHO, are covering up the situation in the Wuhan outbreak. And, if the Chinese government doesn't promote the management to control it, this will become a terrible outbreak or pandemic later. And also, I tell that there is no one animal host—and also the Wuhan seafood market is a smoke screen. And the last thing is, I tell that this is a bioweapon designed by Chinese military lab which is using the backbone of Gaoshan bat coronavirus ZC45 and ZXC21. And also, I released some genomes comparation [meaning? comparison?] like the E protein [indistinguishable] identical proofs through that media. So that makes in China they are scared because they didn't know someone can help this outside.

My winning is to tell the international world because that YouTube blogger based in US maybe there are some foreign audience or young people. And I also maybe some other pressure—at least from international sites—back to China government and lead them to counter this outbreak as soon as possible.

And my work did give the government big pressure, and they respond quickly—just within four hours—to triple the infection—to triple COVID-19 cases from 62 to 198—and then they quickly admit the human-to-human transmission. And also they—at this level of the infectious disease of SARS-CoV-2 [raise] from the nonimportant thing to the SARS1 level— then three days later the government suddenly gave the lockdown order— though this is not my idea. But government thought that is the way to contradict that kind of outbreak. But they still let the people who carry the virus going out and all over the world and later becoming the disaster. And those travelers are innocent—and also, people in the other world are innocent. The thing is the China government locked down Wuhan and locked down other cities but deliberately released these people out. And later I have found several research still in my lab and collaborated with Chinese scientists and has done a lot of research, including publish my *Nature* paper as Cooper's Ulcer using a [indistinguishable] hamster as a transmissional model for COVID-19 animal model—which is a highly recommended paper because for the first time gives the right transmissional model. And the right transmissional model is also the reason China government made a mistake and thought this virus was under their control. So they dared to put it out of the bio safety lab to do their community trial and later make it a disaster. And also the China government because I kept hearing after the news [indistinguishable], and also ITJ 13 is fake. All these things made China government angry. And then they targeted me. At the end of April, I was tranmissional issues—warned by Mr. [indistinguishable] in US, and he said I am in danger. And I have managed to get to US. Because at the same time I noticed the English-speaking country and the Chinese-speaking population are totally isolated. So I also want the Western world to know what really happened. And then I fled to the US. And my family, my friends, all the people who know me, and immediately they become controlled by the government. And, so, I am actually, the kind of enemy to CCP, and they spread a lot of rumor using the media to attack me, and I get a lot of threats. So that is the reason I have to stay in something secret. And also, that is why I publish my three reports in the non–peer reviewed way, because I don't want to delay the time. I don't know want them that they will make me be scared. So at least I can show people the evidence. People like you, and Dr. Fleming, you can read the report, see the evidence, and verify the information for yourselves—even when I am silent or disappeared. So, that is basically the story in short.

Dr. Karladine Graves:
Thank you. We do really appreciate that you have done what you are doing—as well as Dr. Fleming. You are both taking a risk. I think that you know that. I think we all take a risk—all of us who are standing up for the truth and getting it out to the world.

A Gain-of-Function Bioweapon

In 2019, the world was reintroduced to a type of warfare that had previously been made illegal around the world following World War I, when chemical weapons were used to physically maim and destroy soldiers on the battle front. At that time, this type of weapon was thought to be so incomprehensible and appalling that humanity called for its cessation.

History has shown us that evil will raise its ugly head when given the opportunity. The United States has repeatedly demonstrated that even where there is an abundance of the best of humanity, the worst of humanity still dwells. Evil always believes what it is doing is right. Dr. Joseph Mengele thought he was right to conduct research on those he deemed inferior. Unfortunately these types of research projects were carried out long before Mengele, and they have continued long since.

It is said that good men need do nothing for evil to prosper, and history has shown this once again to be the case. The chapters in this book outlined what could have been a positive chapter in human history—a better understanding of these infectious diseases so as to reduce their threat to humanity through research, including how they infect and harm us, as well as how to stop them. Unfortunately, that is not the path many took. Instead, they chose to expose and increase the threat to humanity and in some instances to do so for financial gain.

In the end, the US government funded and developed a bioweapon that was built by the Chinese Communist Party (CCP). It appears that the American government, along with private funders, was playing the Chinese government, and the Chinese government was playing the American government, with the rest of us caught in the crossfire. For this, those who participated in the funding, development, implementation, and firing of this weapon should and must be held accountable for their crimes against humanity.

We have looked at the publication pathway paid for by US federal agencies, including the Department of Defense, Health and Human Services, National Science Foundation, US Agency for International Development, Department of Commerce, Department of Agriculture, Department of the Interior, the National Institutes of Health, and the National Institute of Allergy and Infectious Diseases.

We have seen the patents issued following this research and an accelerated, dangerous release of biologics containing what the evidence shows to be Gain-of-Function sequences assembled by scientists and physicians. The opening of Pandora's box released "exhausting labor, sickness, disease, pain, and death."

In the words of Theognis of Megara[1] from the sixth century BC,

> Hope is the only good god remaining among mankind;
> the others have left and gone to Olympus.
> Trust, a mighty god has gone, Restraint has gone from men,
> and the Graces, my friend, have abandoned the earth.
> Men's judicial oaths are no longer to be trusted, nor does anyone
> revere the immortal gods; the race of pious men has perished and
> men no longer recognize the rules of conduct or acts of piety.

This book opens Pandora's box one last time by revealing what is really happening, who is responsible, and what we can do about it. This time, as with Pandora's final opening of the box, the writing of this book is to release *hope*—hope because we have successful treatments and hope because we have a path to remove from power those who have released this pandemic upon humanity. They are truly responsible for **crimes against humanity** and must be brought to true justice for those crimes!

Despite the power of these people committing crimes against humanity, there are still those among us choosing to expose, sometimes at great cost, what these people have done and continue to do. People like Dr. Li-Meng Yan, who bravely stepped forward to tell the world what she knows. People like Dr. Karladine Graves, who embraced Dr. Yan's and my discussion as we exposed the truth about this Gain-of-Function bioweapon. People like Professor David W. Clements, Del Bigtree, Alex Newman, Dr. Kevin

W. McCairn, Professor Luc Montagnier, Jean-Claude Perez PhD, Pastor Stephen Broden, and a host of other people, who have repeatedly reported on this Gain-of-Function bioweapon and provided a voice for those of us trying to get this important information out to all of you and to call for the criminal accountability of those responsible for violating the Biological Weapons Convention treaty and causing this devastation, destruction, and death across the planet. For my small role in exposing the truth and providing evidence of treatments that work, I am grateful to be associated with these brave, outstanding people. Finally, I would like to thank a special group of people in Dallas, Texas, who embraced the truth and stepped forward when others retreated!

Appendix

Packaged spliced sequences of hepatitis C virus, human inmmunodeficeincy virus-1, SARS-CoV-1, and SARS-CoV-2.[1]

Packaged spliced sequences of HCV (5'-noncoding region, 300nt), HIV-1 (LTR, 331), SARS-CoV1(379 nt), and SARS-CoV2(190 nt).
(Each sequence is started with its name. The positions of primer pair and probe of each sequence are underlined)

HCV

ACACTCCACCATGAATCACTCCCCTGTGAGGAACTACTGTCTTCAC<u>GCAGAAAGCGTC</u>

<u>TAGCCATGGCGT</u>TAGTATGAGTGTCGTGCAGCCTCCAGGACCCCCCCTCCCGGGAGA

GCCATAGTGGTC<u>TGCGGAACCGGTGAGTACA</u>CCGGAATTGCCAGGACGACCGGGTCC

TTTCTTGGATAAACCCGCTCAATGCCTGGAGATTTGGGCGTGCCCCCGCAAGA<u>CTGCT</u>

<u>AGCCGAGTAGTGTT</u>GGGTCGCGAAAGGCCTTGTGGTACTGCCTGATAGGGTGCTTGC

HIV-1

GAGTGCCCCGGGA<u>TTCCAGGGAGGCGTGGCCTGGGCGGGACTGGGGAGTGGCGAGC</u>

CCTCAGATCCTGCATATAAGCAGCTGCTTTTTGCCTGTACTGGGTCTCTCTGGTTA<u>GAC</u>

<u>CAGATCTGAGCCTGGGAGCTCTCTGGCTAACTAGGGAACCCACTGCTTAAGCCTCAAT</u>

<u>AAAGCTTGCCTTGA</u>GTGCTTCAAGTAGTGTGTGCCCGTCTGTTGTGTGA<u>CTCTGGTAA</u>

<u>CTAGAGATCCCTCAGACCC</u>TTTTAGTCAGTGTGGAAAATCTCTAGCAGTGGCGCCCGA

SARS-CoV1

ACAGGGACCTGAAAGCGAAAGGGAAACCAGAGGAGCTCTCTCGACGCAGGACTCGC

TAACATGCTTAGGATAATGGCCTCTCTTGTTCTT<u>GCTCGCAAACATAACACTTGC</u>TGT

AACTTATCACACCGTTT<u>CTACAGGTTAGCTAACGAGTGTGCG</u>CAAGTATTAAGTGAGA

TGGTC<u>ATGTGTGGCGGCTCACTATATGT</u>TAAACCAGGTGGAACATCATCCGGTGATGC

TACAACTGCTTATGCTAATAGTGTCTTTAACATTTGTCAAGCTGTTACAGCCAATGTA

AATGCACTTCTTTCAACTGATGGTAATAAGATAGCTGACAAGTATGTCCGCAATCTAC

AACACAGGCTCTATGAGTGTCTCTATAGAAATAGGGATGTTGATCATGAATTCGTGGA

SARS-CoV2

TGAGTTTTACGCTTACCTGCGTAAACATTT<u>ATGAATTACCAAGTCAATGGTTACCCTA</u>

ATATGT<u>TTATCACCCGCGAAGAAGCT</u>ATTCGTCACGTT<u>CGTGCGTGGATTGGCTTTGA</u>

<u>TGTAGAGGGCTGTCATGCAACTAGAGATGCTGTGGGTACTAACCTACCTCTCCAGCTA</u>

<u>GGATTTTCTACAGGTGTTAACTTAGTAGCTGTACCGACTGGTTATG</u>

The sequences of primers and probes used for RT-PCR detection

HCV
Forward primer: 5'-GCAGAAAGCGTCTAGCCATGGCGT-3'
Reverse primer: 5'-AACACTACTCGGCTAGCAGT-3'
Displacing probes:
  5'-FAM-CTGCGGAACCGGTGAGTACA-PO₄-3'
  5'-TACTCACCGGTTCCGCAG-Dabcyl-3'

HIV-1
Forward primer: 5'-GACCAGATCTGAGCCTGGGAGCT-3'
Reverse primer: 5'-GGGTCTGAGGGATCTCTAGTTACCAGAGT-3'
Displacing probes:
  5'-FAM-CTTAAGCCTCAATAAAGCTTGCCTTGA-PO₄-3'
  5'-AAGGCAAGCTTTATTGAGGCTTAAG-Dabcyl-3'

SARS-CoV1
Forward primer: 5'-GCTCGCAAACATAACACTTGC-3'
Reverse primer: 5'-ACATATAGAGAGCCGCCACACATG-3'
Displacing probes:
  5'-FAM-CTACAGGTTAGCTAACGAGTGTGCG-PO₄-3'
  5'-CACACTCGTTAGCTAACCTGTAG-Dabcyl-3'

SARS-CoV2
Forward primer: 5'-TTATCACCCGCGAAGAAGCT-3'
Reverse primer: 5'-GTAGGTTAGTACCCACAGCATCTCTAGT-3'
Displacing probes:
  5'-FAM-CGTGCGTGGATTGGCTTTGATGTAGAG-PO₄-3'
  5'-CTACATCAAAGCCAATCCACGCACG-Dabcyl-3'

Fleming Inflammation and Heart Disease Theory[2]

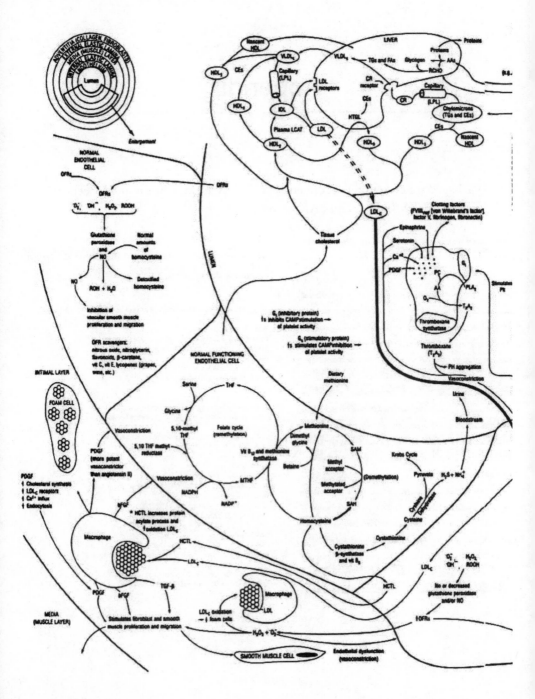

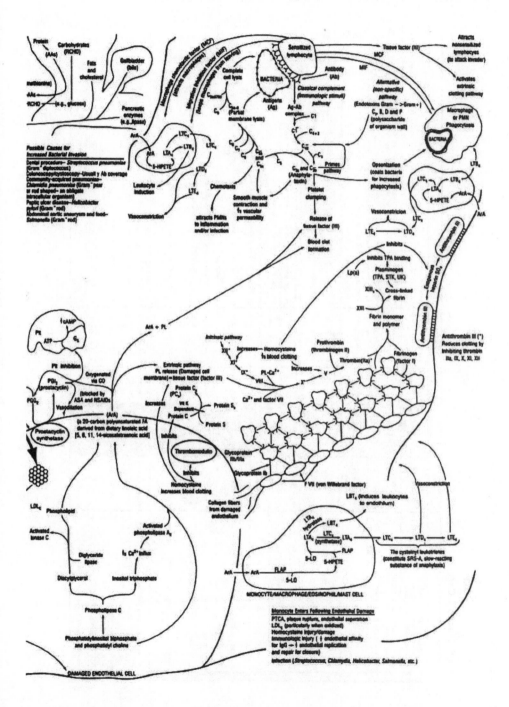

Federal Grant monies paid to Peter Daszak of EcoHealth

Fed. Grants & Contracts

* : Contract Contains Sub Awards

AGENCY	AWARD ID	YEAR	AMOUNT AWARDED	TOTAL AMOUNT	RECIPIENT	DESCRIPTION
Defense Threat Reduction Agency (DOD)	HDTRA11SC0041	2015	$3,217,037.00	$4,479,678.00	ECOHEALTH ALLIANCE	BASE PERIOD - PSC: AD92 IGF-OT-IGF
		2016	$1,262,641.00			
Defense Threat Reduction Agency (DOD)	HDTRA11710027	2017	$721,249.00	$1,604,523.00	ECOHEALTH ALLIANCE	SEROLOGICAL BIOSURVEILLANCE FOR SPILLOVER OF HENIPAVIRUSES AND FILOVIRUSES AT AGRICULTURAL AND HUNTING HUMAN\ANII PENINSULAR MALAYSIA
		2018	$883,274.00			
Defense Threat Reduction Agency (DOD)	HDTRA11910033	2019	$998,437.00	$4,988,987.00	ECOHEALTH ALLIANCE	REDUCING THE THREAT OF RIFT VALLEY FEVER THROUGH ECOLOGY, EPIDEMIOLOGY AND SOCIO-ECONOMICS
		2020	$3,990,550.00			
Defense Threat Reduction Agency (DOD)	HDTRA113C0029 *	2013	$1,371,611.00	$2,225,134.00	ECOHEALTH ALLIANCE	BASE PERIOD
		2014	$957,145.00			
		2015	$108,622.00			
DOD		2014	$892,669.00	$2,942,019.00	ECOHEALTH ALLIANCE	UNDERSTANDING RIFT VALLEY FEVER IN THE REPUBLIC OF SOUTH AFRICA
		2015	$978,794.00			
		2016	$970,556.00			
Defense Threat Reduction Agency (DOD)	HDTRA11410029 (#1)	2017	$996,147.00	$1,994,340.00	ECOHEALTH ALLIANCE	UNDERSTANDING RIFT VALLEY FEVER IN THE REPUBLIC OF SOUTH AFRICA, CHANGE OF ACO TO ONR
		2018	$998,193.00			
Defense Threat Reduction Agency (DOD)	HDTRA11410029 (#2)	2020	$4,912,818.00	$4,912,818.00	ECOHEALTH ALLIANCE	REDUCING THE THREAT FROM HIGH-RISK PATHOGENS CAUSING FEBRILE ILLNESS IN LIBERIA
Defence Threat Reduction Agency (DOD)	HDTRA12010016	2017	$782,330.00	$6,491,025.00	ECOHEALTH ALLIANCE	UNDERSTANDING THE RISK OF BAT-BORNE ZOONOTIC DISEASE EMERGENCE IN WESTERN ASIA
	HDTRA11710064	2018	$2,203,917.00			
		2019	$1,995,247.00			
		2020	$1,509,531.00			
Defense Threat Reduction Agency (DOD)	HDTRA12010018	2020	$4,995,106.00	$4,995,106.00	ECOHEALTH ALLIANCE	CRIMEAN-CONGO HEMORRHAGIC FEVER: REDUCING AN EMERGING HEALTH THREAT IN TANZANIA.
Uniformed Services University of the Health Sciences (DOD)	HU000112010031	2020	$1,360,002.00	$1,360,002.00	ECOHEALTH ALLIANCE	STRATEGIC COORDINATION TO STRENGTHEN AFRICOM ONE HEALTH AND VETERINARY PROGRAMS FOR GLOBAL HEALTH ENGAGEMENT STRENGTHENING MULTI-SECTORAL APPROACHES TO BIODEFENSE AND BIOSURVEILLANCE IN THE CAUCASUS
Defense Threat Reduction Agency (DOD)	HDTRA12010029	2020	$2,956,309.00	$2,956,309.00	ECOHEALTH ALLIANCE	REDUCING THE THREAT OF MIDDLE EAST RESPIRATORY SYNDROME CORONAVIRUS AND AVIAN INFLUENZA IN JORDAN\&STRENGTHENING REGIONAL DISEASE SURVEILLANCE CAPACITY
National Institutes of Health (PHS)	R01TW000S869	2008	$677,758.00	$3,725,160.00	ECOHEALTH ALLIANCE	THE ECOLOGY, EMERGENCE AND PANDEMIC POTENTIAL OF NIPAH VIRUS IN BANGLADESH
		2009	$1,001,885.00			
		2010	$753,006.00			
		2011	$761,334.00			
		2012	$501,437.00			
National Institutes of Health (PHS)	K08AI067549	2008	$100,309.00	$442,844.00	ECOHEALTH ALLIANCE	RISK FOR FUTURE OUTBREAKS OF HENIPAVIRUSES IN SOUTH ASIA
		2009	$110,244.00			
		2010	$118,958.00			
National Institutes of Health (PHS)	R56TW009S002 *	2012	$300,000.00	$300,000.00	ECOHEALTH ALLIANCE	COMPARATIVE SPILLOVER DYNAMICS OF AVIAN INFLUENZA IN ENDEMIC COUNTRIES
National Institute of Allergy and Infectious Diseases (HHS - NIH)	R01AI110964 *	2014	$565,441.00	$3,748,715.00	ECOHEALTH ALLIANCE	UNDERSTANDING THE RISK OF BAT CORONAVIRUS EMERGENCE
		2015	$635,484.00			
		2016	$611,280.00			
		2017	$597,112.00			
		2018	$581,646.00			
		2019	$604,980.00			
CDC OFFICE OF ACQUISITION SERVICES (HHS)	HHSD2002011M41651P	2016	$59,74.00	$99,294.00	ECOHEALTH ALLIANCE	BUSHMEAT
		2018	$45,009.00			
National Institutes of Health (PHS)	R01AI079231	2008	$555,455.00	$2,579,553.00	ECOHEALTH ALLIANCE	RISK OF VIRAL EMERGENCE FROM BATS
		2009	$555,383.00			
		2010	$440,429.00			
		2011	$510,004.00			
		2012	$518,980.00			
NIH NATIONAL INSTITUTE OF ALLERGY AND INFECTIOUS DISEASES (HHS)	U01AI151797	2020	$1,541,744.00	$1,546,744.00	ECOHEALTH ALLIANCE	UNDERSTANDING RISK OF ZOONOTIC VIRUS EMERGENCE IN EID HOTSPOTS OF SOUTHEAST ASIA
Department of Health and Human Services (HHS)	U01AI153430	2020	$580,858.00	$580,858.00	ECOHEALTH ALLIANCE	STUDY OF NIPAH VIRUS DYNAMICS AND GENETICS IN ITS BAT RESERVOIR AND OF HUMAN EXPOSURE TO NIV ACROSS BANGLADESH TO UNDERSTAND PATTERNS OF HUMAN OUTBREAKS

Agency	Office / Program	ID	Year	Amount	Total	Recipient	Project Title
NSF	National Science Foundation (NSF)	1818019	2016 / 2017	$160,233.00 / $309,674.00	$469,897.00	ECOHEALTH ALLIANCE	ECOHEALTH NET 2.0: A ONE HEALTH APPROACH TO DISEASE ECOLOGY RESEARCH & EDUCATION
NSF	NSF	1724994	2017 / 2020	$138,000.00 / $40,150.00	$97,750.00	N/A REDACTED DUE TO PII	DEVELOPING A QUANTITATIVE MODEL OF ECOHEALTH JUSTICE: A CASE STUDY OF MADISON AND MILWAUKEE, WI
NSF	Division of Environmental Biology (NSF)	1015791	2010 / 2012 / 2013 / 2014	$29,109.00 / $13,948.00 / $14,293.00 / $14,652.00	$72,002.00	ECOHEALTH ALLIANCE	COLLABORATIVE RESEARCH: THE COMMUNITY ECOLOGY OF VIRAL PATHOGENS - CAUSES AND CONSEQUENCES OF COINFECTION IN HOSTS AND VECTORS
NSF	NSF	1257513	2012	$22,890.00	$22,890.00	ECOHEALTH ALLIANCE	US-CHINA ECOLOGY AND EVOLUTION OF INFECTIOUS DISEASES COLLABORATIVE WORKSHOP, KUNMING, CHINA - OCTOBER, 2012
NSF	DIVISION OF ENVIRONMENTAL BIOLOGY (NSF)	955897	2010 / 2011 / 2012 / 2013 / 2014	$99,611.00 / $98,673.00 / $99,319.00 / $99,592.00 / $99,936.00	$497,131.00	ECOHEALTH ALLIANCE	ECOHEALTHNET: ECOLOGY ENVIRONMENTAL SCIENCE AND HEALTH RESEARCH NETWORK
NSF	NSF	0622391	2006 / 2008	$303,291.00 / $431,794.00	$932,085.00	ECOHEALTH ALLIANCE	PREDICTING SPATIAL VARIATION IN WEST NILE VIRUS TRANSMISSION
NSF	NSF	0826279	2008	$468,673.00	$468,673.00	ECOHEALTH ALLIANCE	HSD: COLLABORATIVE RESEARCH: HUMAN-RELATED FACTORS AFFECTING EMERGING INFECTIOUS DISEASES
USAID	USAID	AID486A1300005	2013 / 2016	$1,599,203.00 / $899,944.00	$2,499,147.00	ECOHEALTH ALLIANCE	LAND USE CHANGE & DISEASE EMERGENCE
DHS	SCI TECH ACQ DIV (DHS)	70RSAT19C00000012	2019	$566,274.00	$566,274.00	ECOHEALTH ALLIANCE	RAPID EVALUATION OF PATHOGENS TO PREVENT EPIDEMICS IN LIVESTOCK (REPEL) PROJECT TO APPLY BIOLOGICAL-BASED, PATHOGEN AGNOSTIC MEDICAL COUNTERMEASURE VACCINE AND DIAGNOSTIC PLATFORMS TO DEVELOP FOREIGN ANIMAL AND EMERGING ZOONOTIC LIVESTOCK DISEASE VAC
DHS	OFF OF HEALTH AFFAIRS ACQ DIV (DHS)	HSHQDC16C00113	2016 / 2017 / 2018	$271,272.00 / $327,782.00 / $406,902.00	$1,005,956.00	ECOHEALTH ALLIANCE	IGF-OT-IGF GROUND TRUTH
DHS	SCI TECH ACQ DIV (DHS)	70RSAT18C00031001	2017 / 2018 / 2019	$413,761.00 / $246,770.00 / $40,052.00	$700,583.00	ECOHEALTH ALLIANCE	IGF-CLCT-IGF RESEARCH AND DEVELOPMENT SERVICES FOR THE DEPARTMENT OF HOMELAND SECURITY, SCIENCE AND TECHNOLOGY DIRECTORATE, CHEMICAL AND BIOLOGICAL DEFENSE DIVISION FOR PURPOSES OF DEVELOPING A WEB-BASED APPLICATION AND EARLY WARNING SYSTEM FOR GLOBAL INFECTIOUS DISEASE BIO-EVENTS THAT THREATEN THE US VIA INTERNATIONAL TRANSPORTATION NETWORKS.
DOC	EASTERN ACQUISITION DIVISION KANSAS CITY, Department of Commerce (DOC)	DOCWC133D06CN0251	2006 / 2007 / 2008 / 2009 / 2010	$256,120.00 / $263,228.00 / $276,685.00 / $220,700.00 / $225,200.00	$1,241,933.00	ECOHEALTH ALLIANCE	AERIAL SURVEYS OF RIGHT WHALES
USDA	Department of Agriculture (USDA)	09-7100-0209-CA	2008	$143,000.00	$143,000.00	ECOHEALTH ALLIANCE	CONDUCT AN AVIAN INFLUENZE SURVEILLANCE PROGRAM TO DETECT THE OCCURRENCE OF HIGHLY PATHOGENIC H5N1 AVIAN INFLUENZA IN MEXICO.
USDA	Department of Agriculture (USDA)	09-7100-0209-CA	2009	$100,001.00	$100,001.00	ECOHEALTH ALLIANCE	CONDUCT AN AVIAN INFLUENZE SURVEILLANCE PROGRAM TO DETECT THE OCCURRENCE OF HIGHLY PATHOGENIC H5N1 AVIAN INFLUENZA IN MEXICO.
USDA	Animal and Plant Inspection Service (USDA)	0771000237CA	2007	$403,700.00	$403,700.00	ECOHEALTH ALLIANCE	FINANCIAL ASSISTANCE TO PROVIDE THREE WORKSHOPS IN CENTRAL AND SOUTH AMERICA IN SUPPORT OF THE NATIONAL AVIAN INFLUENZA STRATEGIC PLAN.
DOI	Department of the Interior (DOI)	F12AP01208	2012	$154,087.00	$154,087.00	ECOHEALTH ALLIANCE	ECO HEALTH ALLIANCE - GEOMYCES DESTUCTANS, IMPLICATIONS FOR THE MIGRATION OF WHITE-NOSE SYNDROME BAT
DOI	US Fish & Wildlife Services (DOI)	F12AP01117	2012	$44,499.00	$44,499.00	ECOHEALTH ALLIANCE	DEVELOPMENT OF A GREAT APE HEALTH UNIT IN SABAH, MALAYSIA
DOI	US Fish & Wildlife Services (DOI)	F14AP00269	2014	$29,988.00	$29,988.00	ECOHEALTH ALLIANCE	ECOSYSTEM APPROACH FOR BIODIVERSITY MONITORING AND CONSERVATION
DOI	OFFICE OF ACQUISITION AND GRANTS - RESTON (DOI)	IN6G04E5A0526	2004 / 2005 / 2006 / 2007 / 2008	$16,000.00 / $15,000.00 / $10,000.00 / $10,000.00 / $10,000.00	$61,000.00	ECOHEALTH ALLIANCE	04-2070-0909 MANATEE RESSAR
DOI	Department of the Interior (DOI)	G0GAC00002	2011	-$22,512.00	-$22,512.00	ECOHEALTH ALLIANCE	SEABIRD ECOLOGICAL ASSESSMENT NETWORK-SEANET

SUMMARY

FEDERAL GRANTS & CONTRACTS

	AGENCY	TOTAL	
DoD***	Department of Defense	$38,949,941.00	2013-2020
HHS**	Health & Human Services	$13,023,168.00	2007-2020
NSF	National Science Foundation	$2,590,418.00	2006-2020
USAID	U.S. Agency for International Development	$2,499,147.00	2013-2016
DHS	Department of Homeland Security	$2,272,813.00	2016-2019
DoC	Department of Commerce	$1,241,933.00	2006-2010
USDA	U.S. Department of Agriculture	$646,701.00	2007-2009
DoI	Department of the Interior	$267,062.00	2004-2014
GRAND TOTAL			**$61,491,183.00**

** Includes NIH and CDC.
*** Also provided "Policy Advisor" David Franz. Former Commander for Fort Detrick - Principal U.S. Government Bioware/Biodefense Facility.

CHAR500 government grants paid to EcoHealth in 2017: $15,085,333

CHAR500 Schedule 4b: Government Grants (Updated December 2017)

Bushmeat document from the Centers for Disease Control (CDC)

Accessible version: https://www.cdc.gov/importation/bushmeat.html

Bushmeat

What is bushmeat?

* The term "bushmeat" refers to raw or minimally processed meat that comes from wild animals in certain regions of the world including Africa and may pose communicable disease risk.

* Bushmeat comes from a variety of wild animals, including bats, nonhuman primates (monkeys), cane rats (grasscutters), and duiker (antelope).

* Bushmeat is often smoked, dried, or salted (these procedures are not sufficient to render the meat noninfectious).

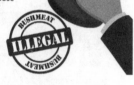

Bushmeat is illegal

* It is illegal to bring bushmeat into the United States.

* Bushmeat, in any amount, found at US ports of entry will be destroyed along with any personal items that may have come in contact with the bushmeat.

* There is a $250,000 fine for bringing bushmeat into the United States.

Bushmeat and Ebola

* Ebola is a rare and deadly disease that is spread through direct contact with the blood or body fluids of a person who is sick with or died from Ebola. www.cdc.gov/vhf/ebola/about.html

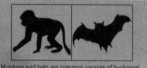
Monkeys and bats are common sources of bushmeat.

* Generally, Ebola is not spread by food. However, in Africa human infections have been associated with hunting, butchering, and processing meat from infected animals.

* To date, there have been no reports of human sickness in the United States from preparing or consuming bushmeat illegally brought into the United States

Health concerns

* Bushmeat could be infected with germs that can cause sickness in people, including the Ebola virus.

* Ebola infections in people have been associated with handling and eating infected animals.

Take action

* Do not bring bushmeat into the United States.

* Do not eat or handle bushmeat.

* Tell friends and family to avoid African bushmeat, because it is illegal to bring it into the United States, and it can make people sick.

* If you must handle bushmeat, wear disposable gloves. When you remove your gloves, wash your hands with soap and water.

* If you choose to eat bushmeat, make sure it is cooked thoroughly.

U.S. Department of Health and Human Services
Centers for Disease Control and Prevention

To learn more about bushmeat, visit:
www.cdc.gov/importation/index.html

You can learn more about the Ebola outbreak in West Africa, visit:
www.cdc.gov/vhf/ebola/index.html

CS298782   December 07, 2018

Homeland Security Office of Health Affairs—National Biosurveillance Integration Center

Homeland Security
Office of Health Affairs
National Biosurveillance Integration Center

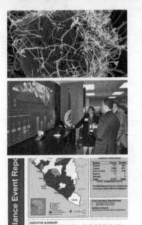

The National Biosurveillance Integration Center (NBIC) integrates and analyzes information about biological threats to help ensure the nation's responses are well-informed, save lives, and minimize economic impact.

Biosurveillance to Protect & Respond

The threat of bioterrorism and the global reach of emerging diseases like Ebola, Foot and Mouth, and Avian Flu require our nation's decision-makers to have timely, accurate and actionable information.

The NBIC is a collaboration of federal partners to integrate information about threats to human, animal, plant, and environmental health from thousands of sources to develop a more comprehensive picture of the threat landscape. The resulting information helps the nation better prepare, protect, and respond.

Mission: Enable early warning and shared situational awareness of acute biological events and support better decisions through rapid identification, characterization, localization, and tracking.

What NBIC Does

- **Integrates information** from various sources and provides an analysis of the likely implications.
- **Monitors and reports** daily on the status of diseases such as chikungunya, enterovirus, the flu, MERS, and Ebola. NBIC also produces periodic analytic reports on special topics and events.
- **Shares** and supports biosurveillance with federal, state, local, tribal, and territorial offices.
- **Improves** biosurveillance by continually seeking innovative data sources and methods.

How NBIC Can Help

- **Monitoring List.** Daily email to partners with brief summaries of global and national biological incidents.
- **Biosurveillance Event Reports.** Comprehensive reports about events that could potentially cause economic damage, social disruption, or loss of life.
- **Special Event Reports.** By request reports, such as a public health assessment for a selected event (e.g. Super Bowl).

NBIC Quick Facts

- **900 federal** and **1500** state and local officials have access to NBIC reports on emerging and current bio-threats.
- **Thousands** of data sources are monitored daily to identify, characterize, and track biological events
- Staffed by cross-discipline **subject matter experts** in public health, veterinary medicine, microbiology, data analytics, and biosurveillance
- Leverages the expertise of **14 federal departments and agencies** to provide a comprehensive and common understanding of emerging incidents
- Federal, state, and local government officials may **request NBIC reports** by emailing NBICOHA@hq.dhs.gov

HealthAffairs@hq.dhs.gov
@DHSHealth1

Source: www.dhs.gov/sites/default/files/publications/2015-Factsheet-NBIC_0 .pdf.

Endnotes

Chapter 1

1. "The Enabling Act: Hitler Seizes Absolute Power," History on the Net, July 21, 2021, https://www.historyonthenet.com/enabling-act-1933.

2. R. M. Fleming, "The Pathogenesis of Vascular Disease," in *Textbook of Angiology*, ed. John C. Chang (New York: Springer Verlag, 1999), 787–98. https://doi.org/10.1007/978-1-4612-1190-7_64.

3. R. M. Fleming, Fleming Method for Tissue and Vascular Differentiation and Metabolism (FMTVDM) Using Same State Single or Sequential Qualification Comparisons. US Patent 9566037, issued February 14, 2017, https://patents.google.com/patent/US9566037B2/en.

4. Comorbities are health problems established prior to SARS-CoV-2 infection and associated with inflammation and blood clotting; some examples are advanced age, obesity, heart disease, a stroke, diabetes, cancer, and high blood pressure.

5. C. Guérin et al, "Prone Positioning in Severe Acute Respiratory Distress Syndrome," *New England Journal of Medicine* 368, no. 23 (2013): 2159–68; Xavier Elharrar et al., "Use of Prone Positioning in Nonintubated Patients with COVID-19 and Hypoxenic Acute Respiratory Failure," *JAMA* 323, no. 22 (2020): 2336–38. doi:10.1001/jama.2020.8255; Acute Respiratory Distress Syndrome Network, "Ventilation with Lower Tidal Volumes as Compared with Traditional Tidal Volumes for Acute Lung Injury and the Acute Respiratory Distress Syndrome," *New England Journal of Medicine* 342, no. 18 (2000): 1301–8; National Heart, Lung, and Blood Institute Clinical Trials Network, "Higher versus Lower Positive End Exxpiratory Pressures in Patients with the Acute Respiratory Distress Syndrome," *New England Journal of Medicine* 351, no. 4 (2004): 327–36.

6. "List of Nazi Doctors," Wikipedia, last updated July 16, 2021, https://en.wikipedia.org/wiki/List_of_Nazi_doctors#:~:text=After%20the%20war%2C%20

the%20German%20Medical%20Association%20blamed,States%20
during%20%22%20Operation%20Paperclip%20%22%20in%201951.

7. "German Medical Association Apologizes for Nazi-Era Experiments," CBS News, May 25, 2012, https://www.cbsnews.com/news/german-medical-association -apologizes-for-nazi-era-experiments/.

8. "Nuremberg Code," Wikipedia, last updated July 20, 2021, https://en.wikipedia .org/wiki/Nuremberg_Code.

9. "The Hunger Games: Hope," YouTube, posted by H. J. M. Edits. Video, 2:47, https://www.youtube.com/watch?v=GkPA4n35-Yk.

10. Complimentary DNA is Reverse Transcription (mRNA reverse transcribed to DNA) frequently using Moloney murine leukemia virus.

11. Chimeras are creations made by combining the genetic code of one organism with that of another; making a new creation. See https://www.scientificamerican .com/article/3-human-chimeras-that-already-exist/?print=true.

12. Boyd Yount et al., "Reverse Genetics with a Full-Length Infectious cDNA of Severe Acute Respiratory Syndrome Coronavirus," *Proceedings of the National Academy of Sciences* 100, no. 22 (October 28, 2003): 12995–13000.

13. Ralph S. Baric, Directional Assembly of Large Viral Genomes and Chromosomes. US Patent 6,593,111, issued July 15, 2003.

14. Wuze Ren et al., "Difference in Receptor Usage between Severe Acute Respiratory Syndrome (SARS) Coronavirus and SARS-Like Coronavirus of Bat Origin," *Journal of Virology* 82, no. 4 (February 2008): 1899–1907; Yuxuan Hou et al., "Angiotensin-Converting Enzyme 2 (ACE2) Proteins of Different Bat Species Confer Variable Susceptibility to SARS-CoV Entry," *Archives of Virology* 155, no. 10 (October 2010): 1563–69, doi: 10.1007/ s00705-010-0729-6.

15. Ibid.

16. United States Department of Health and Human Services, "HHS Will Lead Government-Wide Effort to Enhance Biosecurity in 'Dual-Use' Research," press release, March 4, 2004, https://fas.org/sgp/news/2004/03/hhs030404. html.

17. D. A. Brian and R. S. Baric, "Coronovirus Genome Structure and Replication," *Current Topics in Microbiology and Immunology* 287 (2005): 1–30.

18. Qiuying Huang et al, "Preparation of a Chimeric Armored RNA as a Versatile Calibrator for Multiple Virus Assays," *Clinical Chemistry* 52, no. 7 (July 1, 2006): 1446–48 and Supplement A, doi:10.1373/clinchem.2006.0699710.

19. Ibid, 1447.

20. Vittoria Colizza et al., "Predictability and Epidemic Pathways in Global Outbreaks of Infectious Diseases: The SARS Cast Study," *BMC Medicine* 5, no. 34 (2007): 1–13, doi:10.1186/1741-7015-5-34.

21. Mark Enserink, "Scientists Brace for Media Storm around Controversial Flu Studies," *Science*, November 23, 2011, https://www.sciencemag.org/news/2011

/11/scientists-brace-media-storm-around-controversial-flu-studies; https://www
.newscientist.com/article/mg21128314-600-five-easy-mutations-to-make
-bird-flu-a-lethal-pandemic/?ignored=irrelevant; https://www.scientificamerican
.com/article/next-influenza-pandemic/.

22. "Dual-Use Research of Concern and Bird Flu: Questions & Answers," Centers for
Disease Control, last reviewed May 13, 2019, https://www.cdc.gov/flu/avianflu
/avian-durc-qa.htm.

23. National Institutes of Health, "Panel III: Perspectives of the Proposed HHS
Framework on Funding HPAI H5N1 GOF Research," YouTube. Video:
1:43:59, https://www.youtube.com/watch?v=ZdTRIgrgmn8&t=15s.

24. Taronna R. Maines et al., "Lack of Transmission of H5N1 Avian-Human
Reassortant Influenza Viruses in a Ferret Model," *Proceedings of the National
Academy of Sciences* 103, no. 32 (August 8, 2006): 12121–26.

25. M. Imai et al., "Experimental Adaptation of an Influenza H5 HA Confers
Respiratory Droplet Transmission to a Reassortant H5 HA/H1N1 Virus in
Ferrets," *Nature* 486 (2012): 420–48.

26. "Dual-Use Research," National Institutes of Health, last updated September 3,
2019,https://oir.nih.gov/sourcebook/ethical-conduct/special-research-considerations
/dual-use-research.

27. Lisa Schnirring, "Experts at NIH Meeting Say H5N1 Research Moratorium
May End Soon," Center for Infectious Disease Research and Policy,
December 18, 2012, https://www.cidrap.umn.edu/news-perspective/2012/12
/experts-nih-meeting-say-h5n1-research-moratorium-may-end-soon;
Lisa Schnirring, "Research Moratorium on Modified H5N1 Viruses Ends,"
Center for Infectious Disease Research and Policy, January 23, 2013, https://www
.cidrap.umn.edu/news-perspective/2013/01/research-moratorium
-modified-h5n1-viruses-ends.

28. Y. Yang et al., "Receptor Usage and Cell Entry of Bat Coronavirus HKU4
Provide Insight into Bat-to-Human Transmission of MERS Coronavirus,"
Proceedings of the National Academy of Sciences 111, no. 34 (August 26, 2014):
12516–21.

29. "Doing Diligence to Assess the Risks and Benefits of Life Sciences Gain-of
-Function Research," the White House, September 17, 2014, https://obama
whitehouse.archives.gov/blog/2014/10/17/doing-diligence-assess-risks
-and-benefits-life-sciences-gain-function-research; Donald G. McNeil Jr., "White
House to Cut Funding for Risky Biological Study, *New York Times*, October 17,
2014, https://www.nytimes.com/2014/10/18/us/white-house-to-cut-funding-for
-risky-biological-study.html.

30. Y. Yang et al., "Two Mutations Were Critical for Bat-to-Human Transmission
of Middle East Respiratory Syndrome Coronavirus," *Journal of Virology* 89,
no. 17 (2015): 9119–23.

31. Rai, "SARS COV2 - Identikit di un killer (Identikit of a killer)," YouTube. Video: 9:01, https://www.youtube.com/watch?v=-kt9pVYgqkI.

32. National Science Advisory Board for Biosecurity, *U.S. Government Gain-of-function GOF Deliberative Process and Funding Pause on Selected Gain-of-Function Research Involving Influenza, MERS, and SARS Viruses.* October 17, 2014, http://www.phe.gov/s3/dualuse/documents/gain-of-function .pdf.

33. Talha Burki, "Ban on Gain-of-Function Studies Ends," *Lancet* 18, no. 2 (February 2018): 148–49.

34. Wuhan City Health Committee (WCHCV), *Wuhan Municipal Health and Health Commission's Briefing on the Current Pneumonia Epidemic Situation in Our City 2019*, updated December 31, 2019, and January 14, 2020, http://wjw.wuhan.gov.cn/front/web/showDetail/2019123108989.

35. Qiuying Huang et al, "Preparation of a Chimeric Armored RNA as a Versatile Calibrator for Multiple Virus Assays," *Clinical Chemistry* 52, no. 7 (July 1, 2006): 1446–48, doi:10.1373/clinchem.2006.0699710.

Chapter 2

1. R. A. Flavell et al., "Site-Directed Mutagenesis: Generation of an Extracistronic Mutation in Bacteriophage QßRNA," *Journal of Molecular Biology* 89, no. 2 (October 25, 1974): 255–72.

2. Charles Weissmann, "The End of the Road," *Landes Bioscience* 6, no. 2 (2012): 970194, http://dx.doi.org/10.4161/pri.19778.

3. M. M. Lai et al., "Recombination between Nonsegmented RNA Genomes of Murine Coronaviruses," *Journal of Virology* 56 (1985): 449–56.

4. Kary B. Mullis et al., Process for Amplifying, Detecting, and/or Cloning Nucleic Acid Sequences, US Patent 4,683,195, 21; Tyler Durden, "Caught Red-Handed: CDC Changes Test Thresholds to Virtually Eliminate New COVID Cases among Vaxx'd," ZeroHedge.com, May 23, 2021, https://www.zerohedge.com/covid-19 /caught-red-handed-cdc-changes-test-thresholds-virtually-eliminate-new -covid-cases-among.

5. R. M. Fleming, "The Pathogenesis of Vascular Disease," in *Textbook of Angiology*, ed. John C. Chang (New York: Springer Verlag, 1999), 787–98. doi:10.1007/978-1-4612-1190-7_64.

6. Chronic inflammatory diseases include coronary artery disease (heart disease), cerebral vascular disease (e.g., a stroke), hypertension (high blood pressure), diabetes mellitus (diabetes), obesity, and cancer.

7. *20/20*, April 16, 2004, "Hidden Heart Disease: Could a Simple, Inexpensive Test Save Your Life?," aired April 16, 2004, on ABC; https://rumble.com /vkb7n1-inflammation-and-heart-disease-2020.html.

8. Richard M. Fleming and Matthew R. Fleming, "FMTVDM Quantitative Nuclear Imaging Finds Three Treatments for SARS-CoV-2," *Biomedical*

Journal of Scientific and Medical Research 33, no. 4 (February 8, 2021): 26041–83, doi: 10.26717/BJSTR.2021.33.005443, https://biomedres.us/fulltexts/BJSTR.MS.ID.005443.php.

9. F. Almazán, "Engineering the Largest RNA Virus Genome as an Infectious Bacterial Artificial Chromosome," *Proceedings of the National Academy of Sciences* 97, no. 10 (2000): 5516–21.

10. Ibid.

11. Boyd Yount, Kristopher M. Curtis, and Ralph S. Baric, "Strategy for Systematic Assembly of Large RNA and DNA Genomes: Transmissible Gastroenteritis Virus Model," *Journal of Virology* 74, no. 22 (December 22, 2000): 10600–11.

12. Ibid.

13. Volker Thiel et al., "Infectious RNA Transcribed In Vitro from a cDNA Copy of the Human Coronavirus Genome Cloned in Vaccinia Virus," *Journal of General Virology* 82 (June 2001): 1273–81.

14. MRC-5 cells (aka Medical Research Council cell strain 5) were grown from the lung tissue of a 14-week-old aborted Caucasian male fetus.

15. One method for doing this is called Clusters of Regularly Interspaced Short Palindromic Repeats (CRISPR).

16. Bredenbeek and Rice, 1992; Mandl et al., 1998.

17. Boyd Yount, Kristopher M. Curtis, and Ralph S. Baric, "Strategy for Systematic Assembly of Large RNA and DNA Genomes: Transmissible Gastroenteritis Virus Model," *Journal of Virology* 74, no. 22 (December 22, 2000): 10600–11.

18. Boyd Yount et al., "Reverse Genetics with a Full-Length Infectious cDNA of Severe Acute Respiratory Syndrome Coronavirus," *Proceedings of the National Academy of Sciences* 100, no. 22 (October 28, 2003): 12995–13000.

19. The ability to use reverse transcription to make cDNA from mRNA.

20. Vero E6 cells are a lineage of kidney epithelial cells taken from an African Green Monkey on March 27, 1962.

21. Boyd Yount et al., "Reverse Genetics with a Full-Length Infectious cDNA of Severe Acute Respiratory Syndrome Coronavirus," *Proceedings of the National Academy of Sciences* 100, no. 22 (October 28, 2003): 12995–13000.

22. NCT04349410. Richard M. Fleming and Matthew R. Fleming, "FMTVDM Quantitative Nuclear Imaging Finds Three Treatments for SARS-Cov-2," *Biomedical Journal of Scientific and Medical Research* 33, no. 4 (February 8, 2021): 26041–83, doi: 10.26717/BJSTR.2021.33.005443, https://biomedres.us/fulltexts/BJSTR.MS.ID.005443.php; Canrong Wu et al., "Analysis of Therapeutic Targets for SARS-CoV-2 and Discovery of Potential Drugs by Computational Methods," *Acta Pharmaceutica Sinica B* 10, no. 5 (May 2020): 766–88; Satish Sagar et al., "Bromelain Inhibits SARS-CoV-2 Infection via Targeting ACE-2, TMPRSS2, and Spike Protein," *Clinical and Translational Medicine* 11, no. 2 (February 2021): e281.

23. Liguo Zhang et al., "Reverse Transcribed SARS-CoV-2 RNA Can Integrate into the Genome of Cultured Human Cells and Can Be Expressed in Patient-Derived Tissues," *Proceedings of the National Academy of Sciences* 118, no. 21 (May 25, 2021): e2105968118.

24. Qiuying Huang et al., "Preparation of Chimeric Armored RNA as a Versatile Calibrator for Multiple Virus Assays," *Clinical Chemistry* 52, no. 7 (July 1, 2006): 1446–48 and Supplement A.

25. Commonly known as the People's Revolutionary Government of the Republic of China. Since 2018, it has been superseded and duties transferred to the Kinmen-Matsu Joint Services, the National Development Council, and other ministries for the Executive Yuan (executive branch) of Taiwan.

26. Genome is the entire genetic code of an organism—for example, the SARS-CoV-1 virus.

27. US Department of Health and Human Services, Coronavirus Isolated from Humans, Patent 7,220,852 B1, issued May 22, 2007.

28. US Food and Drug Administration, "In Vitro Diagnostics EUAs—Molecular Diagnostic Tests for SARS-CoV-2," last updated July 19, 2021, https://www.fda.gov/medical-devices/coronavirus-disease-2019-covid-19 -emergency-use-authorizations-medical-devices/in-vitro-diagnostics -euas-molecular-diagnostic-tests-sars-cov-2.

29. Wuze Ren et al., "Difference in Receptor Usage between Severe Acute Respiratory Syndrome (SARS) Coronavirus and SARS-Like Coronavirus of Bat Origin," *Journal of Virology* 82, no. 4 (February 2008): 1899–1907.

30. Yuxuan Hou et al., "Angiotensin-Converting Enzyme 2 (ACE2) Proteins of Different Bat Species Confer Variable Susceptibility to SARS-CoV Entry," *Archives of Virology* 155, no. 10 (October 2010): 1563–69, doi: 10.1007/ s00705-010-0729-6.

31. PRRA is the alphabetic assignment to four amino acids, specifically proline, arginine, arginine, and alanine.

32. Asian-African animal species frequently used by those like Daszak who attempt to explain SARS-CoV-2 as a naturally occurring (zoonotic) virus.

33. Lisa E. Gralinski et al., "Mechanisms of Severe Acute Respiratory Syndrome Coronavirus-Induced Acute Lung Injury," mBio 4, no. 4 (August 6, 2013): e00271-13, doi:10.1128/mBio.00271-13.

34. Ibid.

35. TMPRSS2 is transmembrane protease serine 2. This enzyme, which breaks apart proteins, is found in humans. The gene for TMPRSS2 is found on human chromosome 21. See https://doi.org/10.1006/geno.1997.4845.

36. Xue Han et al., "Structure of the S1 Subunit C-Terminal Domain from Bat-Derived Coronavirus HKU5 Spike Protein," *Virology* 507 (July 2017): 101–9.

37. Y. Yang et al., "Receptor Usage and Cell Entry of Bat Coronavirus HKU4 Provide Insight into Bat-to-Human Transmission of MERS Coronavirus,"

Proceedings of the National Academy of Sciences 111, no. 34 (August 26, 2014): 12516–21.

38. R. M. Fleming, "The Pathogenesis of Vascular Disease," in *Textbook of Angiology*, ed. John C. Chang (New York: Springer Verlag, 1999), 787–98. https://doi.org/10.1007/978-1-4612-1190-7_64.

39. William T. Gibson et al., "ACE 2 Coding Variants: A Potential X-Linked Risk Factor for COVID-19 Disease," *BioRXiv* (April 14, 2020), https://doi.org/10.1101/2020.04.05.026633.

40. Wanbo Tai et al., "Characterization of the Receptor-Binding Domain (RBD) of 2019 Novel Coronavirus: Implications for Development of RBD Protein as a Viral Attachment Inhibitor and Vaccine," *Cellular & Molecular Immunology* 17, no. 6 (June 2020): 613–20.

41. SARS-CoV, now referred to as SARS-CoV-1, was first reported in China in February of 2003. See https://www.cdc.gov/sars/index.html.

42. "Lethal Deception," Rumble.com, April 22, 2021. Video, 1:31:19, https://rumble.com/vfy3xf-lethal-deception.html.

43. Boyd Yount et al., "Reverse Genetics with a Full-Length Infectious cDNA of Severe Acute Respiratory Syndrome Coronavirus," *Proceedings of the National Academy of Sciences* 100, no. 22 (October 28, 2003): 12995–13000; M. M. Becker, "Synthetic Recombinant Bat SARS-Like Coronavirus Is Infectious in Cultured Cells and in Mice," *Proceedings of the National Academy of Sciences* 105, no. 50 (December 2008): 19944–49.

44. V. D. Menachery et al., "A SARS-Like Cluster of Circulating Bat Coronaviruses Shows Potential for Human Emergence," *Nature Medicine* 21, no. 12 (2015): 1508–13.

45. "New SARS-Like Virus Can Jump Directly from Bats to Humans, No Treatment Available," Gillings School of Global Public Health, November 9, 2015, https://sph.unc.edu/sph-news/new-sars-like-virus-can-jump-directly-from-bats-to-humans-no-treatment-available/.

46. That's something Dr. Fauci now denies (see https://twitchy.com/samj-3930/2021/05/11/its-on-dr-fauci-did-not-like-sen-rand-paul-prying-and-asking-questions-about-his-support-for-nih-funding-of-wuhan-lab-watch/), despite the publication acknowledging NIAID funding.

47. V. D. Menachery et al., "Corrigendum: A SARS-Like Cluster of Circulating Bat Coronaviruses Shows Potential for Human Emergence," *Nature Medicine* 22, no. 4 (2016): 446.

48. Gordon Duff, "Documentary Proof: University of North Carolina Generated COVID-19," State of the Nation (website), April 28, 2020, https://stateofthenation.co/?p=12668.

49. V. D. Menachery et al., "A SARS-Like Cluster of Circulating Bat Coronaviruses Shows Potential for Human Emergence," *Nature Medicine* 21, no. 12 (2015): 1508–13, doi:10.1038/nm.3985.

50. Dr. Carlo Urbani was an Italian microbiologist and physician who first identified Severe Acute Respiratory (SARS) viruses and warned the WHO.

51. A = adenine, C = cytosine, G = guanine, T = thymine, and U (not shown here) = uracil.

52. Richard M. Fleming, Unmasking COVID—Part 1 (self-pub., 2020), Kindle, https://www.amazon.com/Unmasking-CoViD-Dr-Richard-Fleming-ebook/dp/B08N5B2KWG.

53. V. D. Menachery et al., "A SARS-Like Cluster of Circulating Bat Coronaviruses Shows Potential for Human Emergence," *Nature Medicine* 21, no. 12 (2015): 1508–13.

54. V. D. Menachery et al., "Corrigendum: A SARS-Like Cluster of Circulating Bat Coronaviruses Shows Potential for Human Emergence," *Nature Medicine* 22, no. 4 (2016): 446.

55. Bill Gates said it would be a "'tragedy' to pass up a controversial, revolutionary gene-editing technology." Article by Kevin Loria April 12, 2018 *Insider*.

56. Janet Levy, "Mengele's Unethical Research Was Part of Existing Beliefs, Practice," *Jerusalem Post*, August 6, 2020, https://www.jpost.com/israel-news/culture/mengeles-unethical-research-was-part-of-existing-beliefs-practice-637682.

57. Y. Yang et al., "Two Mutations Were Critical for Bat-to-Human Transmission of Middle East Respiratory Syndrome Coronavirus," *Journal of Virology* 89, no. 17 (2015): 9119–23.

58. Ibid.

59. C. Calisher et al,, "Statement in Support of the Scientists, Public Health Professionals, and Medical Professionals of China Combating Covid-19," *Lancet* 395 (2020): e42-43.

60. Zoonotic viruses are viruses spread from animals to people. See https://www.cdc.gov/onehealth/basics/zoonotic-diseases.html.

61. Andrew Kerr, "US Researcher with Chinese Ties Admits He Convinced WHO Team That Missing Wuhan Lab Data Was Irrelevant," *Daily Caller*, March 10, 2021, https://dailycaller.com/2021/03/10/who-investigators-wuhan-lab-database-peter-daszak/.

62. Sam Husseini, "EcoHealth Alliance Has Hidden Almost $40 Million in Pentagon Funding and Militarized Pandemic Science," Independent Science News (website), December 16, 2020, https://www.independentsciencenews.org/news/peter-daszaks-ecohealth-alliance-has-hidden-almost-40-million-in-pentagon-funding/.

Chapter 3

1.   Dwight Eisenhower, "Farewell Address," January 17, 1961, YouTube. Video: 16:14, https://www.youtube.com/watch?v=OyBNmecVtdU.

2. "Unethical Human Experimentation in the United States," Wikipedia, last updated July 19, 2021, https://en.wikipedia.org/wiki/Unethical_human _experimentation_in_the_United_States; "Unethical Human Experimentation," Wikipedia, last updated July 13, 2021, https://en.wikipedia.org/wiki/Unethical _human_experimentation.

3. "Guilty as Charged?," FlemingMethod.com, n.d., https://www.flemingmethod .com/thecase.

4. National Science Advisory Board for Biosecurity, *U.S. Government Gain-of-Function Deliberative Process and Research Funding Pause on Selected Gain-of-Function Research Involving Influenza, MERS, and SARS Viruses*, October 17, 2014, http://www.phe.gov/s3/dualuse/Documents/gain-of-function.pdf.

5. Ibid., footnote 1.

6. George Will, "War and Health," UCLA Department of Epidemiology, February 7, 2002, https://www.ph.ucla.edu/epi/bioter/warandhealth.html.

7. "EcoHealth Alliance Inc.," USASpending.gov, n.d., https://www.usaspending .gov/recipient/b4530532-4f85-c249-5fa5-0b86b6cff0ca-C/latest.

8. https://www.usaspending.gov/award/CONT_AWD_HDTRA115C0041 _9700_-NONE-_-NONE.

9. https://www.usaspending.gov/award/ASST_NON_HDTRA11710037_9761.

10. "Scientific Research—Combatting Weapons of Mass Destruction," SAM. gov, n.d., https://sam.gov/fal/05fbd74d0eb74eb3b06d68e38cf605c5/view.

11. https://www.usaspending.gov/award/ASST_NON_HDTRA11710037_9761.

12. Ibid.

13. https://www.usaspending.gov/award/ASST_NON_HDTRA11910033_9761.

14. Ibid.

15. https://www.usaspending.gov/award/CONT_AWD_HDTRA113C0029 _9700_-NONE-_-NONE.

16. Ibid.

17. https://www.usaspending.gov/award/ASST_NON_HDTRA11410029_9700.

18. Ibid.

19. https://www.usaspending.gov/award/ASST_NON_HDTRA11410029_9761.

20. Ibid.

21. https://www.usaspending.gov/award/ASST_NON_HDTRA12010016_9761.

22. Ibid.

23. https://www.usaspending.gov/award/ASST_NON_HDTRA11710064_9761.

24. Ibid.

25. Ibid.

26. http://www.usaspending.gov/award/ASST_NON_HDTRA12010018_9761.

27. Ibid.

28. https://www.usaspending.gov/award/ASST_NON_HU00012010031 _97HW.

29. Ibid.

30. https://www.usaspending.gov/award/ASST_NON_HDTRA12010029_9761.
31. Ibid.
32. "Fort Detrick," Wikipedia, last updated July 20, 2021, https://en.wikipedia.org
    /wiki/Fort_Detrick.
33. https://www.vet.k-state.edu/alumni-events/awards/distinguished/franz.html.
34. https://www.usaspending.gov/award/ASST_NON_R01TW005869_7529.
35. Ibid.
36. Ibid.
37. https://www.usaspending.gov/award/ASST_NON_K08AI067549_7529.
38. Ibid.
39. https://www.usaspending.gov/award/ASST_NON_R56TW009502_7529.
40. Ibid.
41. https://www.usaspending.gov/award/ASST_NON_R01AI110964_7529.
42. Ibid.
43. Ibid.
44. Ibid.
45. https://www.usaspending.gov/award/CONT_AWD_HHSD2002011
    M41641P_7523_-NONE-_-NONE.
46. Ibid.
47. https://www.cdc.gov/importation/bushmeat.html.
48. https://www.usaspending.gov/award/ASST_NON_R01AI079231_7529.
49. Ibid.
50. https://www.usaspending.gov/award/ASST_NON_U01AI151797_7529.
51. Ibid.
52. Ibid.
53. https://www.usaspending.gov/award/ASST_NON_U01AI153420_7529.
54. Ibid.
55. Ibid.
56. Ibid.
57. https://www.usaspending.gov/award/ASST_NON_1618919_4900.
58. Ibid.
59. Ibid.
60. https://www.usaspending.gov/award/ASST_NON_1714394_4900.
61. Ibid.
62. Ibid.
63. Ibid.
64. https://www.usaspending.gov/award/ASST_NON_1015791_4900.
65. Ibid.
66. https://www.usaspending.gov/award/ASST_NON_1257513_4900.
67. Ibid.
68. https://www.usaspending.gov/award/ASST_NON_0955897_4900.
69. Ibid.

70. https://www.usaspending.gov/award/ASST_NON_0622391_4900.

71. Ibid.

72. https://www.usaspending.gov/award/ASST_NON_0826779_4900.

73. Ibid.

74. https://www.usaspending.gov/award/ASST_NON_AID486A1300005_7200.

75. Ibid.

76. https://www.usaspending.gov/award/CONT_AWD_70RSAT19CB0000013_7001
    -NONE--NONE.

77. Ibid.

78. Ibid.

79. https://www.usaspending.gov/award/CONT_AWD_HSHQDC16C00113
    _7001_-NONE-_-NONE.

80. Ibid.

81. Ibid.

82. US Department of Homeland Security, "The National Biosurveillance
    Integration Center Fact Sheet," April 17, 2013, https://www.dhs.gov/publication
    /nbic-one-pager.

83. Ibid.

84. "National Business Inclusion Consortium," National LGBT Chamber of
    Commerce, n.d., https://www.nglcc.org/NBIC.

85. https://www.usaspending.gov/award/CONT_AWD_70RSAT18CB0031001
    _7001_-NONE-_-NONE.

86. Ibid.

87. Ibid.

88. https://www.usaspending.gov/award/CONT_AWD_DOCWC133F06CN0251
    _1330_-NONE-_-NONE.

89. Ibid.

90. https://www.usaspending.gov/award/ASST_NON_08-7100-0206-CA_12K3.

91. Ibid.

92. Ibid.

93. Ibid.

94. https://www.usaspending.gov/award/ASST_NON_07-7100-0237-CA_12K3.

95. Ibid.

96. https://www.usaspending.gov/award/ASST_NON_F12AP01208_1448.

97. Ibid.

98. https://www.usaspending.gov/award/ASST_NON_F12AP01117_1448.

99. Ibid.

100. https://www.usaspending.gov/award/ASST_NON_F14AP00269_1448.

101. Ibid.

102. https://www.usaspending.gov/award/CONT_AWD_ING04ERSA0526
    _1434_-NONE-_-NONE.

103. Ibid.

104. https://www.usaspending.gov/award/ASST_NON_G05AC00002_1434.
105. Ibid.
106. Natalie Winters, "Wuhan Lab Deleted Fauci's NIH and Gain of Function Mentions from Old Web Pages in Early 2021," National Pulse (website), May 15, 2021, https://thenationalpulse.com/exclusive/wuhan-lab-erases-nih-ties-gof -research/.
107. NIAID Ref. No. 2015-33448, 105.

Chapter 4

1. National Center for Biotechnology Information, "Severe Acute Respiratory Syndrome Cononavirus 2 Isolate Wuhan-Hu-1, Complete Genome," July 18, 2020, https://www.ncbi.nlm.nih.gov/nuccore/1798174254.
2. "SARS-CoV Images," Centers for Disease Control, last reviewed October 30, 2020, https://www.cdc.gov/sars/lab/images.html.
3. Fang Li, "Receptor Recognition Mechanisms of Coronaviruses: A Decade of Structural Studies," *Journal of Virology* 89, no. 4 (February 2015): 1954–64.
4. R. M. Fleming et al., "Weight Loss v. Heart Disease: Weight Loss Is Determined by Caloric Intake. Heart Disease Is Determined by Dietary Inflammatory Components. True Quantification of Coronary Artery Disease Measured by AI Using FMTDM," *Archives of Medicine* 10, no. 5 (2018): 3, doi:10.21767/1989-5216.1000284.
5. Michael Greger, "The Inflammatory Meat Molecule," December 13, 2012, NutritionFacts.org. Video: 3:28, https://nutritionfacts.org/video/the -inflammatory-meat-molecule-neu5gc/.
6. M. Jaume, "Anti-Severe Acute Respiratory Syndrome Coronavirus Spike Antibodies Trigger Infection of Human Immune Cells via a pH- and Cysteine Protease-Independent FcγR Pathway," *Journal of Virology* 85, no. 20 (2011): 10582–97.
7. Dapeng Li et al., "The Functions of SARS-CoV-2 Neutralizing and Infection-Enhancing Antibodies In Vitro and in Mice and Nonhuman Primates," *BioRXiv* (February 18, 2021): https://doi.org/10.1101/2020.12.31.424729.
8. Yafei Liu, "An Infectivity-Enhancing Site on the SARS-CoV-2 Spike Protein Is Targeted by COVID-19 Patient Antibodies," *BioRXiv* (December 18, 2020): https://doi.org/10.1101/2020.12.18.423358.
9. J. Shang et al., "Cell Entry Mechanisms of SARS-CoV-2," *Proceedings of the National Academy of Sciences* 117, no. 21 (2020): 11727–34; Indwiani Astuti and Y. Ysrafil, "Severe Acute Respiratory Syndrome Coronavirus 2 (SARS-CoV-2): An Overview of Viral Structure and Host Response," *Diabetes and Metabolic Syndrome* 14, no. 4 (July-August 2020): 407–12.
10. Y. Hou et al., "New Insights into Genetic Susceptibility of COVID-19: An ACE2 and TMPRSS2 Polymorphism Analysis," *BMC Medicine* 18 (2020): 216.

11. S. Bunyavanich et al., "Racial/Ethnic Variation in Nasal Gene Expression of Transmembrane Serine Protease 2 (TMPRSS2)," *JAMA* 324, no. 15 (2020): 1–2.

12. Stacy Malkan, "FOI Documents on Origins of COVID-19, Gain-of-Function Research and Biolabs," USRTK.org, July 9, 2021, https://usrtk.org/tag/ecohealth -alliance/.

13. Ibid.

14. Marcus Hoffman, Hannah Kleine-Weber, and Stefan Pöhlmann, "A Multibasic Cleavage Site in the Spike Protein of SARS-CoV-2 Is Essential for Infection of Human Lung Cells," *Molecular Cell* 78, no. 4 (May 2020): 779–84.

15. Karl Sirotkin and Dan Sirotkin, "Might SARS-CoV-2 Have Arisen via Serial Passage through an Animal Host or Cell Culture?," *BioEssays* 42, no. 10 (October 2020): https://doi.org/10.1002/bies.202000091.

16. Marcus Hoffman, Hannah Kleine-Weber, and Stefan Pöhlmann, "A Multibasic Cleavage Site in the Spike Protein of SARS-CoV-2 Is Essential for Infection of Human Lung Cells," *Molecular Cell* 78, no. 4 (May 2020): 779–84; Li-Meng Yan et al., *Unusual Features of the SARS-CoV-2 Genome Suggesting Sophisticated Laboratory Modification Rather Than Natural Evolution and Delineation of Its Probable Synthetic Route*, New York: Rule of Law Society and Rule of Law Foundation, 2020.

17. Patent Number 7,223,390 B2 issued 29 May 2007 "Insertion of Furin Protease Cleavage Sites in Membrane Proteins and Uses Thereof"

18. S. Hallenberger et al., "Inhibition of Furin-Mediated Cleavage Activation of HIV Glycoprotein gp160," *Nature* 360 (1992): 358–361.

19. Ibid.

20. We will leave the discussions of nonstructural protein 7 (NSP7) and the relationship with the Chinese military for another day. See Aartjan J. W. te Velthuis et al., "The SARS Coronavirus nsp7+nsp8 Complex Is a Unique Multimetric RNA Polymerase Capable of Both De Novo Initiation and Primer Extension," *Nucleic Acids Research* 40, no. 4 (2012): 1737–47.

21. Wuze Ren et al., "Difference in Receptor Usage between Severe Acute Respiratory Syndrome (SARS) Coronavirus and SARS-Like Coronavirus of Bat Origin," *Journal of Virology* 82, no. 4 (February 2008): 1899–1907; Yuxuan Hou et al., "Angiotensin-Converting Enzyme 2 (ACE2) Proteins of Different Bat Species Confer Variable Susceptibility to SARS-CoV Entry," *Archives of Virology* 155, no. 10 (October 2010): 1563–69, doi: 10.1007/s00705-010-0729-6; HA Harrop and CC Rider, "Heparin and its derivatives bind to HIV-1 recombinant envelope glycoproteins, rather than to recombinant HIV-1 receptor, CD4," *Glycobiology* 8, no. 2 (1998):131-137; R Mahfoud R et al., "Identification of a common sphingolipid-binding domain in Alzheimer, prion, and HIV-1 proteins," *J Biol Chem* 277, no. 13 (2002):11292-11296; Y Lu,

DX Liu, JP Tam, "Lipid rafts are involved in SARS-CoV entry into VERO E6 cells," *Biochemical and Biophysical Research Communications* (2008): 344-349; Richard M. Fleming, Unmasking COVID—Part 1 (self-pub., 2020), Kindle, https://www.amazon.com/Unmasking-CoViD-Dr-Richard-Fleming-ebook/dp/B08N5B2KWG; A Bachis A et al., "Human Immunodeficiency Virus Type I Alters Brain-Derived Neurotrophic Factor Processing in Neurons," *J Neurosci* 32, no. 28 (2012): 9477-9484. Supported by AIDS Research and Reference Reagent Program (Dr. R. Gallo, Division of AIDS, NIAID, NIH); RM Fleming RM, MR Fleming, and GM Harrington, "Weight Loss vs. Heart Disease: Weight Loss is Determined by Caloric Intake. Heart Disease is Determined by Dietary Inflammatory Components. True Quantification of Coronary Artery Disease Measured by AI Using FMTVDM," *Arch Med* 10, no. 5 (2018): 3, DOI:10.21767/1989-5216.1000284; RM Fleming, "The Pathogenesis of Vascular Disease" in the *Textbook of Angiology*, Chapter 64, Ed. John C. Chang (New York, NY: Springer-Verlag, 1999), 787-798. doi:10.1007/978-1-4612-1190-7_64.

22. Ibid.

23. Ibid.

24. Yuxuan Hou et al., "Angiotensin-Converting Enzyme 2 (ACE2) Proteins of Different Bat Species Confer Variable Susceptibility to SARS-CoV Entry," *Archives of Virology* 155, no. 10 (October 2010): 1563–69, doi: 10.1007/s00705-010-0729-6.

25. Ibid.

26. Dr. Shi Zhengli is also known as Dr. Shi Zhengli-Li, depending upon the published material.

27. Y. Yang et al., "Two Mutations Were Critical for Bat-to-Human Transmission of Middle East Respiratory Syndrome Coronavirus," *Journal of Virology* 89, no. 17 (2015): 9119–23.

28. National Science Advisory Board for Biosecurity, *U.S. Government Gain-of-Function Deliberative Process and Research Funding Pause on Selected Gain-of-Function Research Involving Influenza, MERS, and SARS Viruses*, October 17, 2014, http://www.phe.gov/s3/dualuse/Documents/gain-of-function.pdf.

29. Wuze Ren et al., "Difference in Receptor Usage between Severe Acute Respiratory Syndrome (SARS) Coronavirus and SARS-Like Coronavirus of Bat Origin," *Journal of Virology* 82, no. 4 (February 2008): 1899–1907.

30. A molecule combined of both a carbohydrate and protein.

31. L. Du et al., "The Spike Protein of SARS-CoV—a Target for Vaccine and Therapeutic Development," *Nature* 7 (2009): 226–36.

32. B. J. Bosch et al., "The Coronavirus Spike Protein Is a Class I Virus Fusion Protein: Structural and Functional Characterization of the Fusion Core Complex," *Journal of Virology* 77, no. 16 (2003): 8801–11.

33. "Lethal Deception," Rumble.com, April 22, 2021. Video, 1:31:19, https://rumble.com/vfy3xflethal-deception.html.

34. Prashant Pradhan, "Uncanny Similarity of Unique Inserts in the 2019-nCoV Spike Protein to HIV-1 gp120 and Gag," *BioRXiv* (February 2, 2020): https://doi.org/10.1101/2020.01.30.927871.

35. Chengxin Zhang et al., "Protein Structure and Sequence Re-Analysis of 2019-nCoV Genome Does Not Indicate Snakes as Its Intermediate Host or the Unique Similarity between Its Spike Protein Insertions and HIV-1," *BioRXiv* (February 8, 2020): https://doi.org/10.1101/2020.02.04.933135.

36. Ibid.

37. "Lethal Deception," Rumble.com, April 22, 2021. Video, 1:31:19, https://rumble.com/vfy3xflethal-deception.html.

38. "Luc Montagnier," Wikipedia, last updated July 21, 2021, https://en.wikipedia.org/wiki/Luc_Montagnier.

39. J. C. Perez and L. Montagnier, "COVID-19, SARS, and Bats Coronaviruses Genomes Peculiar Homologous RNA Sequences," *International Journal of Research* 8, no. 7 (July 2020): 217–63.

40. J. C. Perez and L. Montagnier, "COVID-19, SARS and Bats Coronaviruses Genomes Unexpected Exogenous RNA Sequences," https://www.researchgate.net/publication/341756383.

41. Ibid.

42. J. C. Perez and L. Montagnier, "COVID-19, SARS, and Bats Coronaviruses Genomes Peculiar Homologous RNA Sequences," *International Journal of Research* 8, no. 7 (July 2020): 217–63.

43. A codon is a three nucleotide sequence. Each codon codes for a specific amino acid. Therefore, each three nucleotide sequence (codon) codes for a specific amino acid.

44. J. C. Perez and L. Montagnier, "COVID-19, SARS, and Bats Coronaviruses Genomes Peculiar Homologous RNA Sequences," *International Journal of Research* 8, no. 7 (July 2020): 217–63.

45. Li-Meng Yan et al., "The Wuhan Laboratory Origin of SARS-CoV-2 and the Validity of the Yan Reports Are Further Proved by the Failure of Two Uninvited "Peer Reviews," http://www.researchgate.net/publication/350523980; Li-Meng Yan et al., *Unusual Features of the SARS-CoV-2 Genome Suggesting Sophisticated Laboratory Modification Rather Than Natural Evolution and Delineation of Its Probable Synthetic Route*, New York: Rule of Law Society and Rule of Law Foundation, 2020, md5:95dd4b8062a82f09779e39f5bbb7a487.

46. "Severe Acute Respiratory Syndrome (SARS)–Corona Virus (CoV) 2, from Infection to COVID-19. Treatments and Vaccines," FlemingMethod.com, n.d., illustration, https://www.flemingmethod.com/documentation.

47. Electronic Support for Public Health—Vaccine Adverse Event Reporting System (ESP:VAERS). Submitted to AHRQ Grant Final Report. Grant ID: R18 HS 017045.

48. "Death and Mass Injury from the Swine Flu Vaccine of 1976, Back when *60 Minutes* Did Their Job," Bitchute.com, May 17, 2021. Video: 14:31, https://www.bitchute.com/video/0lFlz0WzgU3r/.

49. "Guillain-Barré Syndrome Fact Sheet," National Institutes of Health, n.d., https://www.ninds.nih.gov/Disorders/Patient-Caregiver-Education/Fact-Sheets/Guillain-Barr%C3%A9-Syndrome-Fact-Sheet.

50. R. M. Fleming, "The Pathogenesis of Vascular Disease," in *Textbook of Angiology*, ed. John C. Chang (New York: Springer Verlag, 1999), 787–98, doi:10.1007/978-1-4612-1190-7_64.

51. Ibid.

52. Dominic Wichmann et al., "Autopsy Findings and Venous Thromboembolism in Patients With COVID-19," *Annals of Internal Medicine* (August 18, 2020): doi:10.7326/M20-2003.

53. J. Bart Classen, "Review of COVID-19 Vaccines and the Risk of Chronic Adverse Events Including Neurological Degeneration," *J Med - Clin Res & Rev* 5, no. 4 (2021): 1-7.; J. Bart Classen, "COVID-19 RNA Based Vaccines and the Risk of Prion Disease," *Microbiol Infect Dis* 5, no. 1 (2021): 1-3; Jenny Meinhardt et al., "Olfactory Transmucosal SARS-CoV-2 Invasion as a Port of Central Nervous System Entry in Individuals with COVID-19," *Nature Neuroscience* 24 (2021): 168–75, https://doi.org/10.1038/s41593-020-00758-5; Elizabeth M. Rhea et al., "The S1 Protein of SARS CoV-2 Crosses the Blood-Brain Barrier in Mice," *Nature Neuroscience* 24 (2021): 368–78, https://doi.org/10.1038/s41593-020-00771-8; Mariano Carossino et al., "Fatal Neuroinvasion of SARS-CoV-2 in K18-hACE2 Mice Is Partially Dependent on hACE2 Expression," *BioRXiv* (January 15, 2021): https://doi.org/10.1101/2021.01.13.425144; Ingrid H. C. H. M. Philippens et al., "SARS-CoV-2 Causes Brain Inflammation and Induces Lewy Body Formation in Macaques," *BioRXiv* (May 5, 2021): https://doi.org/10.1101/2021.02.23.432474.

54. K. Bahl et al., "Preclinical and Clinical Demonstration of Immunogenicity by mRNA Vaccines against H10N8 and H7N9 Influenza Viruses," *Molecular Therapy* 25, no. 6 (2017): 1316–27.

55. Mariano Carossino et al., "Fatal Neuroinvasion of SARS-CoV-2 in K18-hACE2 Mice Is Partially Dependent on hACE2 Expression," *BioRXiv* (January 15, 2021): https://doi.org/10.1101/2021.01.13.425144.

56. Ingrid H. C. H. M. Philippens et al., "SARS-CoV-2 Causes Brain Inflammation and Induces Lewy Body Formation in Macaques," *BioRXiv* (May 5, 2021): https://doi.org/10.1101/2021.02.23.432474.

57. L. Jiao et al., "The Olfactory Route Is a Potential Way for SARS-CoV-2 to Invade the Central Nervous System of Rhesus Monkeys," *Signal Transformation and Targeted Therapy* 6 (2021): 169, https://doi.org/10.1038/s41392-021-00591-7.

58. Ingrid H. C. H. M. Philippens et al., "SARS-CoV-2 Causes Brain Inflammation and Induces Lewy Body Formation in Macaques," *BioRXiv* (May 5, 2021): https://doi.org/10.1101/2021.02.23.432474.

59. R. M. Fleming et al., "The Importance of Differentiating between Qualitative, Semi-Qualitative and Quantitative Imaging–Close Only Counts in Horseshoes," invited editorial, *European Journal of Nuclear Medicine and Molecular Imaging* 47, no. 4 (2020): 753–55, doi:10.1007/s00259-019-04668-y, published online January 17, 2020, https://link.springer.com/article/10.1007/s00259-019-04668-y.

60. "Lewy Body," Wikipedia, last updated July 21, 2021, https://en.wikipedia.org/wiki/Lewy_body.

61. Rossana Segreto et al., "An Open Debate on SARS-CoV-2's Proximal Origin Is Long Overdue," https://www.researchgate.net/publication/349125078.

62. J. B. Classen, "Review of COVID-19 Vaccines and the Risk of Chronic Adverse Events Including Neurological Degeneration," *Journal of Medical-Clinical Research & Reviews* 5, no. 4 (2021): 1–7.

63. S. Seneff and G. Nigh, "Worse Than the Disease? Reviewing Some Possible Unintended Consequences of the mRNA Vaccines against COVID-19," *International Journal of Vaccine Theory, Practice, and Research* 2, no. 1 (2021): 402–43.

64. A biological is a diagnostic, pregentive, or therapeutic deived or obtained from living organisms and their product, including serum, vaccine, antigen, and antitoxin.

65. "Severe Acute Respiratory Syndrome (SARS)–Corona Virus (CoV) 2, from Infection to COVID-19. Treatments and Vaccines," FlemingMethod.com, n.d., illustration, https://www.flemingmethod.com/documentation.

66. Karen O'Hanlon Cohrt, "How to Calculate the Number of Molecules in Any Piece of DNA," Bitesize Bio, https://bitesizebio.com/20669/how-to-calculate-the-number-of-molecules-in-any-piece-of-dna/; "Reverse Engineering the Source Code of the BioNTech/Pfizer SARS-CoV-2 Vaccine," December 25, 2020, https://berthub.eu/articles/posts/reverse-engineering-source-code-of-the-biontech-pfizer-vaccine/.

Chapter 5

1. "Biological Weapons Convention," United Nations, n.d., https://www.un.org/disarmament/biological-weapons.

2. "Biological Weapons," Office of the Law Revision Counsel, n.d., https://uscode.house.gov/view.xhtml?path=/prelim@title18/part1/chapter10&edition=prelim.